The Post-Pandemic World and Global Politics

AKM Ahsan Ullah · Jannatul Ferdous

The Post-Pandemic World and Global Politics

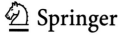

AKM Ahsan Ullah
Faculty of Arts and Social Sciences
Universiti Brunei Darussalam
Gadong, Brunei Darussalam

Jannatul Ferdous
Comilla University
Cumilla, Bangladesh

ISBN 978-981-19-1909-1   ISBN 978-981-19-1910-7   (eBook)
https://doi.org/10.1007/978-981-19-1910-7

© The Editor(s) (if applicable) and The Author(s), under exclusive license to Springer Nature
Singapore Pte Ltd. 2022
This work is subject to copyright. All rights are solely and exclusively licensed by the Publisher, whether
the whole or part of the material is concerned, specifically the rights of translation, reprinting, reuse
of illustrations, recitation, broadcasting, reproduction on microfilms or in any other physical way, and
transmission or information storage and retrieval, electronic adaptation, computer software, or by similar
or dissimilar methodology now known or hereafter developed.
The use of general descriptive names, registered names, trademarks, service marks, etc. in this publication
does not imply, even in the absence of a specific statement, that such names are exempt from the relevant
protective laws and regulations and therefore free for general use.
The publisher, the authors and the editors are safe to assume that the advice and information in this book
are believed to be true and accurate at the date of publication. Neither the publisher nor the authors or
the editors give a warranty, expressed or implied, with respect to the material contained herein or for any
errors or omissions that may have been made. The publisher remains neutral with regard to jurisdictional
claims in published maps and institutional affiliations.

This Springer imprint is published by the registered company Springer Nature Singapore Pte Ltd.
The registered company address is: 152 Beach Road, #21-01/04 Gateway East, Singapore 189721,
Singapore

Preface

The Covid-19 pandemic has had a profound effect on people's lives worldwide, touching every aspect of society. This means that the world has been experiencing a global health crisis, with governments implementing a variety of mitigation strategies, including halting the spread of the virus, stabilizing healthcare systems, and securing employment and businesses. Some institutions, such as government, education, and business, responded in ways that enabled the Virus to spread and have varying effects depending on area, colour, ethnic origin, gender, and socioeconomic class.

Pandemic preparations and responses have been impacted by politics since it was a public health and political crisis. Nevertheless, a connection between global health issues and political issues is still being established. There have been many system-level connections between governments and health epidemics and infectious diseases since the eighteenth century, such as cholera, small pox and Typhus and Yellow Fever and the Bubonic Plague.

This book reveals how assumptions regarding the origins, consequences, and reactions to the COVID-19 outbreak are addressed via the prism of politics and the diverse perspectives of experts in this field. This book aims to generate recommendations for more research into critical components of global politics in the COVID-19 era as it develops and advances from and for scholars studying global politics.

The COVID-19 pandemic has had a significant impact on domestic politics, affecting the governance and political systems of most of the countries, suspending legislative activity, isolating or killing politicians, rescheduling elections, and prohibiting protests due to fears of the Virus spreading. However, several governments exploited the outbreak as an excuse to prohibit political activities. As a result, the pandemic has spawned broader political debates regarding the relative merits of democracy and autocracy, as well as how governments respond to crises. The pandemic has precipitated an economic crisis, with job losses exceeding job increases over the preceding decade in a matter of months and wreaking havoc on several areas of life.

The majority of the world powers seemed to be concerned about the origin of the Virus. Some politicians instigate conspiracy theories and disseminate fake information regarding the Virus's origins. Such speculative assertions may serve only to divert attention away from researchers and policy makers working to contain the Virus's spread. The question is: Is it worthwhile to continue a raging debate over the origins of Covid-19, or should we instead concentrate on applying what we have learned and planned for the future?

Politicizing the epidemic has resulted in the emergence of anti-vaxxers. Vaccine refusal is a significant factor in the continued rise in COVID-19 infections. The bulk of these folks belongs to the right-wing political parties. Despite health professionals' urge that vaccination is an issue of public health, not politics, they continue to say COVID-19 is a scam.

Not all of our concerns about the global politics-pandemic nexus have been answered by this book, but it does highlight how politicians may explain away the reality and hence tend to perpetuate the pandemic.

Gadong, Brunei Darussalam   AKM Ahsan Ullah
Cumilla, Bangladesh   Jannatul Ferdous
2022

Contents

1 The Pandemic and Global Politics 1
  Introduction 1
  The Politics of the Origin-Trace 3
  Argument, Objectives and Methods 6
  Political Geography of the Pandemic 9
  Reshaping Democratic Space 11
  A New World Order 13
  Health Regime and Governance 15
  Organization of the Book 16
  Conclusions 17
  References 18

2 Underlying Conceptual Approach: An Era or a Crisis? 23
  Introduction 23
  The Origin Theory Discourse 28
  The Foundation of Crisis Models 31
  Pandemic Governance and Security Approach 40
  Digital Divide and Growing Disparity 41
  Conclusions 44
  References 46

3 Politicization of Pandemic and the Ramifications 53
  Introduction 53
  What the History Has to Tell Us 55
  Reshaping Compliance 60
    Cooperation and Compliance 61
  Political Temperature and Responses 65
    Africa 68
    Latin America 69
    Asia 71
  The Migration Domain 71
  The Public Health 73

viii   Contents

Disparity	76
Gender	79
Education	82
Discrimination	84
Citizen Trust	86
Politics of Anti-masks and Anti-vaccines	88
Conclusions	94
References	95

4 Pandemic, Predictions and Propagation 105

Introduction	105
The Economic Landscape	108
Politics and Electoral System	113
Freedom of Expression	116
Prejudice and Sigma	118
Security for Women	120
Citizen Trust	123
The Future Globalization	124
The Health Care System	127
Education and Digitalization	129
Interdependence	131
The Gainers and the Losers	133
Getting Ready for the Future	134
Reopening Plans	138
Conclusions	140
References	143

5 Choosing to End the Pandemic: Conclusions and Discussion 153

Introduction	153
Is everything Going to Change?	155
Implications for Politics	158
The Recovery Plans	169
Is resilience the Only Option?	169
Let's Not This Pandemic Go To Waste	172
References	174

About the Authors

AKM Ahsan Ullah is Associate Professor in Geography, Environment and Development at the University of Brunei Darussalam (UBD). Dr. Ullah's research portfolio includes stints at the Southeast Asian Research Centre (SEARC), Hong Kong; University of Ottawa, McMaster University; Saint Mary's University, and Dalhousie University, Canada; the American University in Cairo (AUC); City University of Hong Kong, Hong Kong, Osnabruck University, Germany, and Asian Institute of Technology (AIT), Thailand. His research areas include population migration, human rights, development, environment and health policy. Dr. Ullah has contributed 60 scientific articles to refereed journals and at least 40 chapters in a number of books, and published 15 books.

Jannatul Ferdous is Associate Professor, Department of Public Administration, Comilla University, Bangladesh. Dr. Ferdous received her bachelor, masters and M.Phil. in Public Administration from the University of Dhaka. Dr. Ferdous contributed extensively to refereed journals and chapters in books. She published seven books. Her current interest includes governance, e-governance, trust, civil service system, gender, public policy, climate change, gender and development. Currently, she is serving as the Chair of the technical committee of the 'Combating Gender-Based Violence' project of UN Women. She is also serving as an assistant proctor of Comilla University.

Abbreviations

ASEAN	The Association of Southeast Asian Nations
BRICS	Brazil, Russia, India, China, & South Africa
CDC	Centers for Disease Control and Prevention
COVID	Coronavirus Disease
EIP	European Institute of Peace
GBV	Gender Based Violence
GDP	Gross Domestic Product
GGP	Governance Global Practice
GVC	Global Value Chains
HIV	Human Immunodeficiency Virus
HRW	Human Rights Watch
ICG	International Crisis Group
ILO	International Labour Organization
IMF	International Monetary Fund
MERS	Middle East Respiratory Syndrome
MFAPRC	Ministry of Foreign Affairs of the People's Republic of China
MSME	Ministry of Micro, Small & Medium Enterprises
OECD	Organisation for Economic Co-operation and Development
PAP	People's Action Party
SAARC	South Asian Association for Regional Cooperation
SARS	Severe Acute Respiratory Syndrome
SSA	Sub-Saharan Africa
UNCTAD	United Nations Conference on Trade and Development
WHO	World Health Organization

List of Figures

Fig. 2.1   The interplay between COVID-19 and global politics (*Sources* Developed by authors based on Arendt, 2020; Bhattacharya & Khan, 2021; Bodrud-Doza et al., 2020; Donnelly et al., 2021; Kishi, 2021; Loayza, 2020; Melvin et al., 2020; Nwankwo, 2021; Obrenovic et al., 2020; Shammi et al., 2021; UNAIDS, 2020; Walby, 2021; WHO, 2020; World Bank, 2021) 42

Fig. 3.1   Share of COVID-19 vaccine by income group (*Source* World Bank, 2021) 64

Fig. 3.2   Anti-vaccine rating (*Source* Woodward, 2021) 93

Fig. 4.1   COVID-19 estimated impact on developing Asian economies (*Source* Sawada & Sumulong, 2021 [with permission]) 112

Fig. 4.2   Election held and postponed during COVID-19 (*Source* International Institute for Democracy and Electoral Assistance [IDEA], 2021 [with permission]) 115

List of Tables

Table 3.1	Estimated reduction in global and regional remittances flow ...	73
Table 3.2	Percentage of death reported in males due to COVID-19 in major countries (Mid 2020)	81
Table 4.1	Estimated job and wage income losses due to COVID-19	109
Table 4.2	Estimated job and wage income losses due to COVID-19 (GDP)	111

Chapter 1
The Pandemic and Global Politics

Introduction

COVID-19 stole 28 million years of life from only 31 countries in 2020 (Gale, 2021), with Russia experiencing the highest decline in life expectancy, with males experiencing 2.33 years and females 2.14 years at birth. The United States ranked second, with males losing 2.27 years and women losing 1.61 years. Bulgaria, Lithuania, Chile, and Spain were the countries to experience a decline in life expectancy (Jeong, 2021). Throughout the research, consolidation of data and writing of the book, we were repeatedly questioned, either by others or ourselves, why write about a pandemic at a time when there is a pandemic. Is there anything else we can do other than focus on the difficult work of dealing with the current situation? Something appears to be lacking from the global discourse about COVID-19. The outbreak consumed our attention for over two years, as far as we were concerned. We discussed the Virus itself, its impact on our lives, and the vaccines. We thought the immunizations that may allow us to return to some kind of normalcy has been well debated. However, we have not discussed nearly enough about the underlying political developments in the domestic, regional, and international spheres. Unfortunately, as we can see, people are dying, and we appear to be so helpless and powerless to stop them. We are so tiny as compared to the might of the Virus.

Lockdowns shut down facilities and forced large segments of the workforce to work from home. Zoom achieved a daily meeting participants peak of over 300 million up from 10 million in December 2019. Their estimate of "annualised meeting minutes" has more than doubled, from 100 billion in late January to more than two trillion in April 2020 (Wired, 2020). In a study for the University of Southern California's Schaeffer Center for Health Policy and Economics, Hanke Heun-Johnson and Bryan Tysinger investigated the equation for all unexpected fatalities that have occurred since the pandemic began (Bump, 2022). The Centres for Disease Control and Prevention uses a statistic called "excess deaths" to compare the number of fatalities documented in the United States to the anticipated number of deaths based

© The Author(s), under exclusive license to Springer Nature Singapore Pte Ltd. 2022
AKM. A. Ullah and J. Ferdous, *The Post-Pandemic World and Global Politics*,
https://doi.org/10.1007/978-981-19-1910-7_1

on prior year's patterns. Heun-Johnson and Tysinger estimate that the additional fatalities have resulted in a loss of 13.5 million years of human life (Bump, 2022).

The primary goal of the book is to help readers make sense of unpleasant events and build a discourse that leads to a future that we all desire. At some point in our lives, we have all felt as if we were in the midst of a hurricane. The breakout of the COVID-19 Virus has flipped the world upside down and radically impacted the way we live. The pandemic has had an impact on all of us in different ways. Certainly, COVID-19 has been a major factor in the tragedy of 2019–2021. Nonetheless, we believe that the underlying cause extends well beyond that. It is well known that people of colour and the poor live shorter and sicker lives than their white counterparts throughout the world. People who live in run-down locations with mould-infested walls fall ill faster. Some people can work from home in the suburbs during a pandemic, while others are obliged to deal with crowds every day at a low-wage job they are frightened of losing. When COVID-19 hit, there was a dearth of assistance for those in need due to a lack of investment in a social safety net in most countries. Amid this disaster, the pandemic became politicized, preventing us from unifying around a shared cause.

A confluence of social, economic, environmental, and political issues has resulted in a world that is no longer as healthy as it should be. COVID-19 set a fire under an already smouldering tinderbox of poor health in our society as a result of the pre-pandemic conditions. While the fire of the pandemic was catastrophic in many ways, it was distinct from a real fire in one crucial sense- the speed of the spread. The true fire eventually consumes the conditions that caused it to start in the first place. Because of the same factors, COVID-19 is no less likely to become a firestorm now than it was in the summer of 2019. All that is required to revive the flames of injustice and misalignment in our society is a fresh spark.

The COVID-19 pandemic is caused by a one-of-a-kind Coronavirus for which science and technology found no immediate cure, and that this Virus has already had a tremendous impact worldwide (Rahman et al., 2021; Ullah et al., 2021). COVID-19, like past pandemics, has altered human history, and it is not an unexpected outcome. Despite examples such as the Black Death (1347–1352), the Third Cholera Pandemic (1852–1860), the Flu Pandemic (1889–1890), and the Influenza (Spanish Flu) pandemic (1918–1920), historians have tended to underestimate the disruptive potential of such diseases in the modern industrialized world (Byrne, 2012; Gottfried, 1983; Hays, 2005; Ranger & Slack, 1992; Snowden, 2020).

The purpose of the introduction is to orient the reader to the research presented in the body of the book. The introduction includes the information necessary to prepare the reader, to put the reader in the picture in terms of the specifics of the research: what this book focuses on; the context of the study, the research questions or objectives driving the investigation, the argument we intend to present, and the book structure. This chapter is meant to highlight the enormity of the impact of COVID-19 on global politics. The most astonishing characteristic of this pandemic is its lethality, which has claimed the lives of millions of people worldwide. It has put into question the efficacy of our scientific and technical advancements. We humans, who once thought of ourselves as world conquerors, are now confined to the boundaries of our dwellings. The adage "time is unpredictable" appears to be true in every sense

Introduction

in today's reality. The COVID pandemic has influenced worldwide collaboration, making COVID-19 a focal point of global politics. The definition of superpower has evolved as they appear impotent in the face of the Virus. States that can deal with COVID-19, on the other hand, are redefining what it means to be a superpower. All of this has fueled fears of a new Cold War, with China and the US playing prominent roles this time. The last cold war was centred on the USSR and the United States, but today, COVID-19 seems to be changing the course of international politics.

The high number of individuals who die as a result of pandemics in developed countries shakes our trust in modern medical sciences. When a pandemic causes a large-scale demographic collapse, relative factor pricing, such as labour vs. land or capital, may be affected. This has the potential to cause enormous changes in the economic and political structures. Differences in factor prices are widely acknowledged to influence economic inequality (Piketty, 2014), which influences both the prevalence of democracy (Acemoglu & Robinson, 2012) and the quality of democratic representation (Bartels, 2008)—despite the notion that factor prices are social structure axis, establishing how they affect political life empirically can be difficult. Relative factor prices influence and are moulded by the public policy because they limit the bargaining power of social groups (Beramendi & Christopher, 2008). Political institutions, which govern public policies, are analogous (Acemoglu, 2010).

COVID-19 has vividly revealed both the cooperating and conflicting components of the world political landscape (Benton, 2018; Bowman & Kearney, 2007). Contacts between states show concern that their breadth has expanded while problematic intergovernmental interactions are not new (Burke & Brudney, 2018). Leaders gained both praise (i.e. New Zealand) and condemnation (i.e. India, Bangladesh, Brazil, USA) as they responded in a variety of ways as the crisis unfolded. Some governments opted for aggressive and visible responses to the pandemic, and some were condemned for the lack of preparedness and slow response (Goodman et al., 2021; Luscombe, 2020; Turner, 2020). State politics and policy, intergovernmental relations, and global politics shape how states can respond to COVID-19. State and local government responses to COVID-19 bring up new scholarly avenues by highlighting mechanisms that are not completely understood in the current models.

The Politics of the Origin-Trace

The frequent mutation of COVID-19 variants has led to a shifting global pandemic at the time, and prevention and control remain extremely challenging all over the world. While the world fights the disease tenaciously, a few countries seem to be focusing on political maneuvering on the COVID-19's origin rather than internal epidemic prevention (MFAPRC [Ministry of Foreign Affairs of People's Republic of China], 2021). The investigation on the origin of the Virus quickly devolves into a political farce as it seemed to disregard and oppose the scientific method. Tracing the origins of viruses is a crucial and challenging scientific task. Its purpose is to prevent and respond to such public health disasters more effectively in the future. It, however, must be accomplished without being politicized or affected by ideologies.

According to the Chinese government, the US intended to politicize the pandemic and stigmatize the Virus from the outset (MFAPRC, 2021). The United States publicly referred to COVID-19 as the "Wuhan Virus" and withdrew from the World Health Organization. It even disregards scientists' efforts by soliciting the assistance of the scientific community to conduct origin-tracing and hype up the so-called lab-leak theory, which is predicated on a presumption of guilt. China terms it shifting blame onto China for the inability to tackle the Virus and achieve the political mileage of undermining China. The WHO Secretariat opted to focus the Phase II origin study on the assumption that "China broke laboratory processes and caused virus leakage," which experts considered was highly unlikely. According to the government, more than 55 countries have approved the China-WHO joint study report on origin-tracing and condemned its politicization (Muurlink & Taylor-Robinson, 2020; Global Times, 2021).

The Chinese government has underlined the necessity of international cooperation in tracing the origins of the Virus. The Chinese position is that mysteries could be solved through open collaboration between countries, and the study of virus genesis should be conducted from a global perspective by scientists from a broader region. Although the Chinese government claims to have been the first to warn the rest of the world about the epidemic, there is no scientific evidence that COVID-19 originated in China.

A never-before-seen storm of political, social, economic, and epidemiological forces was unleashed when the COVID-19 pandemic broke out. The COVID-19 outbreak has had far-reaching political consequences. Policymakers have faced a high-profile issue, balancing the need to stop the Virus from spreading while restarting the economy. A better understanding of COVID-19 has brought the world to ask and answer the question: "Why did some countries do so much worse with regards to coping with COVID-19 (Greer et al., 2021). The COVID-19 epidemic put international pressure on governments to respond quickly. Their policy responses, on the other hand, varied greatly from country to country. Some administrations/governments enacted strict lockdown policies quickly (e.g. Argentina or Australia). Others selected adaptable measures to lessen the economic burden of the pandemic (e.g. Japan, Sweden, Brazil, or the US). Recently, there has been much debate concerning the 'health vs. economics' trade-off (Alvarez et al., 2020). Nonetheless, there is still a scarcity of comprehensive research on how the public reflects on diverse policy responses across multiple countries and over several months.

The pandemics have the capacity to reshape a worldwide discourse about the merits of autocracy vs. democracy. In any pandemic situation, keeping democracy healthy is a big challenge. The Coronavirus is expected to change the essence of democratic government, such as election procedures, civilian control of the military, and civic mobilization. In fact, much is still up in the air, including the ultimate scope and severity of the pandemic (Brown et al., 2020). As the pandemic spreads to low-income and vulnerable countries, the repercussions would undoubtedly be far more deadly and unpredictable than those observed so far. The pandemic certainly has massive consequences on governance by overburdening countries' essential governance duties, stressing their sociopolitical cohesion, worsening corruption, disrupting interactions between local and national governments, and changing the role of non-state actors.

The state becomes an increasingly important and unique component in the fight against pandemics as COVID-19 and other pandemics become widespread and are incorporated into national security frameworks as a perceived reproach. Hence the pandemic will underline the need for strong states. The government is the sole provider of healthcare, security, and welfare during global and national epidemics. As a result of the epidemic, some of the most influential players in the COVID-19 global community found themselves in a bad situation.

This pandemic has afforded us to see that traditional methods of evaluating state power are insufficient for determining the power of the state. When measuring state power, the conventional method frequently misses healthcare systems, supply chains, and emergency service capabilities in addition to military might, economic power, and population. According to some assessments, strong governments may not need to become authoritarian; the assumption that authoritarian regimes are more effective at resisting COVID-19 than democratic states is incorrect, as countries like Germany, Turkey, Japan, South Korea, and others have demonstrated (Ulutaş, 2020) their incapacity to handle the pandemic efficiently. The global epidemic has hit top Western countries hard, and they are revisiting their external threat hierarchy and their international policy priorities.

In recent years, the widely held notion that Russia is the "primary problem" in international relations and the "major threat" to Western interests has been weakening. Given the high cost of multinational projects, such a conceptual shift will likely result in immediate and beneficial improvements in Moscow's ties (for example, implementing the Paris Climate Agreement). The consequences for Russia's "national brand" would be severe if the country's current socioeconomic model is maintained in the post-crisis world. If the existing socioeconomic model in Russia survives the post-crisis world, the ramifications for the country's "national brand" might be devastating (Kahf, 2020).

COVID-19 invades our health and threatens our life in such a way that it damages our spiritual and internal serenity, replacing it with concerns, sorrow, dread, and doubt. These repercussions have affected our social fabric individually, with serious political, economic, social, and cultural ramifications (Torreblanca, 2020). Every international crisis has ramifications for international structures, rules, and institutions. For example, the September 11 terrorist attacks changed global state and law toward non-state individuals. The global financial crisis of 2008 altered the G20 from a council of finance ministers to just a party able of soft steering in a number of less contentious areas of international affairs (Perthes, 2020). The COVID-19 outbreak of 2020 has hastened the recent atomization of international civilization. Global institutions have continued to deteriorate, and international rule-based governance has become increasingly weakened. Multilateralism had devolved into a form of competitive unilateralism. Alliance politics sucked up more goodwill than they produced practical cooperation. Even when many regions went into various degrees of lockdown, several armed confrontations remained.

The outbreak will have long-term geopolitical consequences. International distrust and mistrust are on the rise, and confidence is on the decline. Some states' strategic adventurism further shakes the status quo. The world will be thrown into even more strategic turmoil. Diplomatic and security problems will regularly arise, with sporadic and ineffective attempts to address them. As 2020 ended, specific themes emerged that would shape the international situation in 2021 and later, putting states and institutions under increased strain (IISS, 2020).

While the COVID-19 outbreak has had a greater effect on economic growth than any recent shock, the geopolitical consequences could be much more destructive. In the post-COVID-19 world, a fundamental shift in the international political economy may have been on the horizon. This shift may be dependent on two variables: the first is the extent to which countries afflicted by the pandemic have recovered economically, and the second is the wide range of domestic political possibilities in many countries involved. Before the pandemic, populism—and its extreme authoritarian inclinations, which see the nation-state emerge as a reaction to multilateral-globalist sequence—increased. The most perplexing concern is whether the COVID-19-inspired and widely accepted sense of "we all need each other" will allow for increased global climate change consequences, nuclear arms, global migration, extreme poverty, and biodiversity loss. The implementation of lessons learned outside of health, such as the rate and depth of changes in the healthcare sector, is a good example, would depend on whether more worldwide and future-oriented leadership arises (Eiran, 2020).

Argument, Objectives and Methods

The COVID-19 pandemic has evolved into much more than a global health emergency. It has sparked a worldwide cultural war, shattered the foundations of the healthy functioning of the global economy, highlighted the weakness of the UN system, and driven societies all over the world into fear of an uncertain future.

The world economic crisis and severe acute respiratory symptoms—none have become as severe, long-lasting, or wide-ranging as this current pandemic. The sub-Saharan region would be the most affected by hunger crisis, contributing to 40–50 percent of global poverty growth. Given the significance of India, a major but largely closed economy, an unexpected trade would have a higher impact on Africa's impoverished than on those in South Asia because Africa's economy is more dependent on global commerce on average than those in South Asia. On the other hand, productivity shocks would have a stronger impact on poverty in South Asia than in Africa, owing to the greater negative impact on non-agricultural industries, which are more important in South Asian countries (Vos et al., 2020). Unlike previous crises, it has simultaneously affected the world's leading economies, paralyzed international links, and raised doubts about its eventual abolition. Surprisingly, no effective global response has been triggered for a global turmoil like this incident. Instead, countries have taken various measures based on the costs of virus prevention versus financial closure and isolation.

The lack of evident single world power or the continuous tensions between two top rivals—the United States and China—could explain the absence of global leadership (Enderwick & Buckley, 2020). Tensions among the United States and China, sparked by COVID-19 and violence in other locations, have spurred several issues hurting the unity and solidarity of the global South. Nationalism and populism have become critical variables in the growth and collaboration of emerging countries in the South, not just in the United States and wealthier countries in the North. Most countries will be forced to choose sides if they become politicized, affecting technology transfer, international business and investment, and economic assistance between poor and growing economies. This means that the pandemic has provided most countries with the opportunity to increase or decrease international cooperation (Mohan, 2020). Fortunately, during the COVID-19 outbreak, many countries in the development cooperation sector and the global South showed consistent multilateralism and collaboration. Notably, several southern countries began to send humanitarian aid to industrialized countries as well as other developing countries (Zhou et al., 2020).

Under this backdrop, we try to portray how global politics has taken shapes and how the politicization of the pandemic impacts global health equity. We look into how global and health politics would likely look like in the post-COVID period.

This book is based on a study conducted between March 2020 and August 2021. For this work, we mostly depended on empirical information and the existing research available in various outlets. Between mid-February 2020 and mid-March 2021, we conducted 107 informal interviews (via Skype and WhatsApp) with migrant populations living or stuck in Singapore, Brunei, Hong Kong, Macau, Italy, Spain, Maryland, New York, Newark, Florida, Atlanta, Ohio), Dusseldorf (Germany), Amsterdam (Netherlands), Copenhagen (Denmark), Italy, France, Qatar, Kuwait, and Saudi Arabia. The snowball method was used to choose these respondents.

The historical setting, the pattern of political changes, history of conflicts, and relationship with epidemic and leadership are critically analyzed in this study to locate an intersection between politics, pandemic and leadership. We conducted qualitative research and heavily relied on secondary data sources to better understand how the pandemic has influenced global politics. We painstakingly examined the literature we chose and conducted content analysis (both conceptual and relational). The conceptual analysis finds concepts in the text, whereas the relational analysis builds on the conceptual analysis by examining the connections between concepts. Secondary sources include scholarly books, journal papers, previous surveys, and web sources.

COVID-19 has left world politics with a number of pressing and significant problems. In the wake of the unprecedented global health catastrophe, the US ex-President, Mr. Trump likened it to a struggle with an "invisible adversary," and the British media has compared it to the "spirit of the blitz," a reference to WWII (Williams, 2020). The global status of some particular countries, especially Britain and its key international relationships, have become a pressing priority in this uncertain environment because of Prime Minister's recent key speeches on future trading relations with superpowers such as the United States and China, as well as by the contentious decisions regarding Huawei's access to the phone network in the UK. These two superpowers were already vital for the UK government after Brexit, but the outbreak has made that relationship even more critical.

In terms of economic destruction, the COVID-19 outbreak is unquestionably one of the most devastating ones in history, possibly surpassing the 2008 financial crisis. When it comes to great countries, the disease and its repercussions pose a particularly significant risk. Many giant companies and global leaders have been put at risk by this crisis, underlining their reputation and abilities. The aftermath of the Pandemic might fundamentally alter global political order, with countries rising and sliding in prominence due to its massive effects. Previously significant international events, such as the onset of the Cold War following World War II, had a significant impact. Some have claimed that the shrinking distance between the United States and China could be wiped out in the wake of these catastrophic events. This would be somewhat ironic given the pandemic's origin debate (Williams, 2020). In early 2020, news of an outbreak of the Virus in a Chinese city shocked the world, but no one expected it to spread so quickly. The scientific community has been on high alert, researching the Virus, the disease it causes, the scenario it develops, and the population it attacks from a number of viewpoints, including systematic evaluations of the literature, such as the one presented in this book.

Biology and medicine are not the only fields of study in which this research can be applied. For example, Maestre's (2020), notes that "virus" in Latin means "poison," and hence most current research is focused on finding medicine that will destroy the Virus. Pharmacists are constantly searching for substances that protect people's health or desire for safety (Hall & Prayag, 2020). Participants and communities play an important role in the design and conduct of participatory research. With today's socially divided pandemic environment, participatory tactics rely significantly on creating trust and maintaining personal relationships, becoming increasingly difficult. The preceding concerns are even more crucial (Ullah & Azizuddin, 2018). According to Warner-Mackintosh (2020), wealth, social capital, and access to healthcare (which is increasingly given digitally) and protected information are linked. There are currently a wealth of COVID-19-related publications that focus on content rather than methodology. Participatory research methods have been and could be adapted to the current social condition, with an emphasis on how rapport and equality can be maintained at a distance—both digitally and analogically (Hall et al., 2021).

The COVID-19 outbreak is causing unavoidable changes in every aspect of life, from the social to the economic. Many countries have implemented regulations like "social separation" and "stay-at-home" in reaction to the gravity of the pandemic, which has led to a major shock to businesses and production, even bigger than the Great Depression and World War II (Donthu & Gustafsson, 2020; Piccarozzi et al., 2021).

Narrative reviews and summaries have been impetuously conducted in our literature analyses. The narrative reviews helped us to identify gaps or discrepancies in the body of knowledge. This sort of literature review and assessment necessitates greater precision and rigour than the majority of the others. Different types of systematic literature reviews include meta-analysis and meta-synthesis (De Mauro et al., 2016; Sassanelli et al., 2019). In a meta-analysis, multiple research data are combined and analyzed using established statistical methods. However, meta-synthesis relies on non-statistical methods. In order to support or disprove an established argument, deep-rooted premise, or philosophical quandary, an argumentative literature review selectively examines facts. Prejudice is a basic problem in argumentative literature analysis. In order to provide fresh frameworks and perspectives on an issue under study, an integrated literature review provides analysis and synthesis of secondary sources. An integrated literature review has been our sole choice. Theoretical literature reviews focus on a certain subject, concept, theory, or phenomenon and the resulting body of knowledge. Studies of theoretical literature are useful in determining whether concepts already exist, how they are connected, how thoroughly they have been explored, and in coming up with new testable hypotheses.

Political Geography of the Pandemic

There was only one continent where COVID-19 had not spread until December 2020: Antarctica. As COVID-19 has already reached, the wildlife and ecosystem were at risk. (Sawada & Sumulong, 2021). For a long time after the initial appearance and rapid spread of the Virus globally in early 2020, there was a great deal of skepticism around the Virus's long-term health impact, and it was widely considered that international cooperation would be critical to ending the threat and supporting economic recovery (Beirne et al., 2021; Sawada & Sumulong, 2021). Economic recovery in 2021 is expected to be facilitated by the ultimate distribution of COVID-19 vaccinations, which can help to restore the entire global economy.

The rise of digitalization and remote working is expected to continue, as is digitalization in other economic sectors. COVID-19 is expected to substantially impact economic output in the global COVID map of the world, of course, with varying degrees in different countries. As a result of the pandemic, it is possible that the GDP trend would swing in the opposite direction from pre-pandemic times. Hence, global authorities are now discussing strategies to boost economic resilience, including increasing efforts to promote environmental sustainability and the development of a greener economy. In general, East Asian economies are expected to have suffered slightly less from the COVID-19 Virus because of the aggressive testing and contact tracing that has helped contain domestic outbreaks without the need for strict lockdown measures. Lockdowns implemented in various countries and across borders to stop the virus' spread have had a severe negative economic impact on emerging Asian economies in general (Beirne et al., 2021).

The United States since the beginning of the outbreak has been blaming China for exporting and spreading this deadly Virus around the world. The US blames that China produced COVID-19 on purpose in order to gain dominance and accused the World Health Organization (WHO) of siding with China. The tensions between the United States and China have worried the whole world. Both are the world's most powerful countries, and the conflict might throw civilization back millennia, unleashing disaster. Many political analysts consider this the beginning of a new Cold War (Ashford & Kroenig, 2020). In contrast, Zachary Karabell (2020) projected that there would be no new Cold War with China and that only time would tell who was right about their notion.

Today, the Sino-India relationship reached at an "extremely tough moment" (Feng, 2021), and the relationship between India and China appears to have suddenly grown quite critical. Though both India and China have long experience fighting diseases over their ancient histories (Liu, 2020). The tridimensional conflict [between the US and China and between India and China] created a serious threat to the peaceful coexistence of nations in international affairs. The main sources of conflict between India and China are border conflicts and attacks against armies. As a result of these tensions, the Indian government has declared that Chinese Apps will be banned in India by June 2020. These clashes have strained their bilateral relationship. Both countries seek to strengthen their relationships with other countries to safeguard their interests. The most pressing question is why a border battle turned essential when both countries are battling with the COVID-19 crisis.

The most evident fact is that the race between the US and China will become more intense. In recent decades, American foreign policy has been influenced by the flawed notion that China's economic integration with the West will lead to political improvements, making it a non-threatening partner for large democracies. Even before the current situation, the American foreign policy elites realized that this assumption was a pipe dream. Even before the outbreak, Donald Trump's "maximum pressure" campaign, as well as the wave of political unrest that swept the country in November 2020, had put the government in a legal bind. And, Iran appears to be taking advantage of America's hesitancy. On the other hand, Iran lacks the necessary capacity to fill the gap. Iran, however, seems to emerge from the coronavirus outbreak in a situation of serious deterioration.

Due to the fact that the delta variant originated in India, many people referred to this variant by the place of the origin (i.e. the Indian variant). Scientists and policymakers fear that these labels would be used to stigmatize and punish countries only for the reasons for their emergence (Mueller, 2003). It is worth mentioning that India has retained the term "Wuhan virus" for the Coronavirus. Powell (2012) says that President Joe Biden established a series of COVID-19 protocols in response to the new omicron strain. Although the guidelines/restrictions will have a minimal effect on health, this is not their purpose. Rather than that, these restrictions teach Americans to tolerate increased government intrusions into our lives while eroding the liberty in the name of security (Powell, 2012). Before announcing the restrictions, Biden had barred travel from South Africa, where the omicron strain was found, and seven other south African countries (when such prohibitions were deemed racist).

Political Geography of the Pandemic

The newly announced requirements include an extension of the federal mask requirement for public transportation, including airplanes, until mid-March and requiring international travelers to the United States, including vaccinated Americans, to show proof of a negative COVID-19 test taken the day before departure (Powell, 2012).

It is expected that once the Virus goes under control, life would return to "normal," especially if the vaccine is widely available, administered and distributed without discrimination. It will be difficult to predict the specifics, but there will undoubtedly be some long-term alterations in demand structure. People in advanced economies may work from home for an extended period of time, if not permanently, reducing their need for autos and gasoline. There may be a decrease in the demand for industrial and commercial space. Commodity prices and market volume would likely fall as a result of these developments. Demand will rise for automobiles, electronics, and clothes are three businesses with vast value chains. There should be more demand for gadgets and less for automobiles and clothing in a post-pandemic society. However, the fundamental argument is that substantial shifts in these areas could impact development opportunities. International tourism, a significant export for many developing nations, may not entirely rebound to its prior level in terms of services.

Reshaping Democratic Space

The pandemic is creating a surge in executive power around the world, which has far-reaching implications for democratic space. Since the beginning of the pandemic, most countries have implemented limits on public meetings and freedom of movement and speech. Over fifty countries have proclaimed emergencies (ICNPL, 2021). There are already hints that some governments are exploiting the crisis to award themselves more sweeping powers than the health emergency permits, with inadequate accountability processes, and to stifle opposition and solidify their dominance. As a result, the epidemic can deepen repression in closed political systems, accelerate democratic backsliding in failing democracies, and strengthen executive power inside democratic countries (Brown et al., 2020).

The COVID-19 epidemic is one of the worst disasters humanity has ever faced in the twenty-first century. There appears to be no end in sight. Amidst, in the post-COVID-19 era, political rivalries among world powers, particularly the United States and China, could lead to many disorders (Akon & Rahman, 2020). Brown and his colleagues (2020) have illustrated the connected areas of fear generating new emergency regulations and limits. The government's credibility has been harmed further by its slow response to the coronavirus outbreak. Because of Iran's growing vulnerability, the US will be able to put it on the defensive even without a significant military commitment. The COVID-19 conundrum will reinvigorate nationalism while undermining international institutions such as European Union. Throughout Europe, populist groups have risen in recent years, demanding complete independence from Brussels. This trend is expected to be exacerbated by the outbreak. The global technocrats were of little use in the response to the crisis. Each country was forced to rely on its resources when it mattered most, and this is not simply a European phenomenon, either (Noury et al., 2021; Doran, 2020).

Power consolidation: In the face of a crisis, illiberal leaders strive to cement their authority by removing checks, restrictions, and accountability structures. A new law in Hungary, for example, empowers Viktor Orbán to rule by decree indefinitely without the need for legislative approval. The Philippines President Rodrigo Duterte has signed legislation giving him practically unrestricted emergency powers. Similarly, Cambodia's proposed national emergency plan would grant the government unrestricted martial authority while severely restricting citizens' democratic rights.

Fundamental rights compromised: Some governments are already infringing on citizens' fundamental rights as a result of their emergency powers. Under the pretext of combatting the Virus, one particular tendency is on the increase in the propaganda from individuals who exercise control over freedom of speech and the media about the number of infections. Evidences are rife that journalists who covered the outbreak were arrested, and in many countries, information on the Chinese government's response was restricted. Citizens and the media in many countries such as Bangladesh and India who oppose the government's approach face legal consequences and official intimidation.

State surveillance widened: As a result of this dilemma, governments are increasingly deploying substantial monitoring tools on citizens. Governments are using smartphone location data in Israel and South Korea, for example, to seek down residents who may have been exposed to the Virus. The epidemic has provided another rationale for authoritarian governments to employ increasingly intrusive measures such as widespread social media surveillance and facial recognition. Let us remember the recent controversy around deploying Pegasus spyware to monitor the activities of civilians in many countries. Bangladesh has purchased Israeli surveillance equipment capable of tracking people's smartphones at once (Ritzen, 2021). Newcomers in Hong Kong are forced to wear electronic destination bracelets, whereas Singapore conducts intensive contact tracking and publishes detailed information on every known case. While increased surveillance is not necessarily anti-democratic, there is a huge risk of political abuse if these additional measures are accepted and implemented without transparency or accountability. For example, in India, the government has pressured local media to maintain a positive image despite implementing uncomfortable policies. Using location monitoring to guarantee that the photo was taken at the individual's home is one strategy for requiring solitary folks to post selfies frequently. In Bangladesh, media is tightly controlled by the government. Pro-government journalists and media outlets enjoy the freedom to propagate against the opposition. However, pro-opposition journalists are arrested, and media outlets get closed.

Protests banned: The epidemic of COVID-19 has evidently aggravated a global democratic crisis. Since the outbreak of the pandemic, the health of democracy and human rights has deteriorated in 80 countries (Freedom House, 2020). Many countries have prohibited protests as a pretext for suppressing the recent surge in anti-government marches that have roiled global politics. After significant protests in 2020 that pushed the government to make minimal political concessions, Algerian authorities have ruled all gatherings, marches, and demonstrations illegal. One point to consider is whether these restrictions will be in place indefinitely. Another issue is that it is discriminatory, prohibiting anti-government protests while allowing or encouraging pro-government marches. Governments have retaliated by silencing critics and weakening or shutting down critical organizations, frequently jeopardizing the very accountability structures necessary to protect public health. Since mid-March 2020, the Bangladesh government has imprisoned at least a dozen people, including doctors, opposition activists, and students, for their views about the Coronavirus (Repucci & Slipowitz, 2020).

A New World Order

COVID-19 has thereby exposed the vulnerability of nation-states and the present world order. COVID-19 may have exacerbated a troubling trend toward state isolationism and expedited the erosion of the global governance system and supply chains. The political and economic divide between the United States and China has been uncomfortably exposed as well (Wintermeyer, 2020).

During the 2008 financial crisis, the phrase "new normal" was coined to describe the enormous economic, cultural, and social shifts that resulted in precariousness and social unrest, influencing collective perspectives and individual lifestyles. During the COVID-19 epidemic, this phrase again emphasized how it has changed the fundamental parts of human life (Jeff, 2021). We have been forced to adjust to the 'new normal' a year after the COVID-19 pandemic broke out: work-from-home environments, parents, home-schooling their children in a new blended learning environment, lockdown and quarantine, and the mandated wearing of face masks in public (Jeff, 2021; Ullah et al., 2021). The forced transition to virtual work has resulted in a massive shift in virtual activities. Many of these shifts are fueled by the ostensibly systemic incapacity to successfully respond to the government, economic, and societal crises (Wintermeyer, 2020).

Humanity must prepare for this new "world" that has resulted from the aggressive spread of the Virus and its impact. Containing the epidemic and dealing with the inevitable collateral damage to the world's socioeconomic and political infrastructure should involve politicians and the general people all across the world. Experts, IR and security research academics endeavour to examine the problem or the policy options adopted to handle it. Non-traditional intelligence workers delve further into international health security systems, especially the global disparities in standards. IR specialists in the Global South confront a considerably more difficult role due to the region's low levels of development, population density, resource depletion, poverty, and climatic circumstances, as the pandemic's impact will be far more entrenched and long-lasting (Fazio et al., 2021; Ferdous & Ullah, 2022). Once the Virus has passed by, a new world order may leave its imprint on humans in every part of the world. As governments work together to rebuild the global socioeconomic and political infrastructure, competition and rivalry between them may be subdued. We believe that the habit of maintaining social distance and technologically dependent communication will persist, cross-border trade would continue in a pleasant manner around the world, and the need for international political-economic partnership would be highlighted more than ever before.

Today, we came to realize that the fights against Coronavirus seems to be more complicated than we assumed. Military weapons are useless and inapplicable. We assume that the outbreaks might have served as a wake-up call to bridge the North–South divide by illustrating how they could manage the adversity through information and resource sharing. Setting goals is easier than carrying them out—i.e. de-escalation of the conflict, followed by reconciliation and global action through the formation of a global government alliance. Society becomes more inward-looking as a result of social distancing policies. If humanity is to survive, the Post-COVID economic system needs to be well-managed. It is important that we apply the theoretical insights of the experts in international relations to the new conditions of a 'Coronized' world (Pal, 2020).

Until the collapse of the Soviet Union, it was totally a closed country. It started to open in 1991. Today, Russia's leadership has recently highlighted the supremacy of national government. So far, the epidemiologic issue has supported Russia's position: the crisis strengthens national states. They expose the intergovernmental community's inefficiency and raise doubts about the West's devotion to its stated goals and principles. This initiative expands, for example, Russia's domestic and international propaganda options, bolstering the Kremlin's goal to play a vital role in the post-crisis global order (Trent & Schnurr, 2018).

Under this current situation, it became clear about the necessity of sovereignty while also questioning the stability of Western deployments and the utility of Western pluriliteral negotiation. The global pandemic has dramatically affected the most developed Western countries as well, forcing them to reconsider their external threat hierarchy. As a result, their foreign policy objectives have shifted. In recent decades, Russia has been widely seen as the "chief problem" in international affairs and the "primary threat" to Western interests; however, COVID-19 is swiftly debunking this notion.

The ramifications for Russia's "national brand" will not be any less severe if its current socioeconomic paradigm survives the post-crisis world (Kahf, 2020). The COVID-19 outbreak highlighted our growing interconnection and the urgent need for it at a time when excitement for global collaboration is still in short supply. With the pandemic causing a global recession worth $10 trillion or about 10% of global GDP (Economist, 2021), the world will be unable to respond to present and future crises unless more international solid structures are developed.

In a complex, networked, and panicky world, fundamental alterations in how people work, interact and think have occurred as a result of the escalating US–China race for global leadership. New forms of collaboration and civil rights movements evolved during the COVID-19 era, as did the need for a new kind of national politics. Significant and small countries are currently circling the wagons, which is the polar opposite of the approach needed to combat transnational existential threats to human health and the environment (Carayannis & Weiss, 2021).

Health Regime and Governance

Technology, economics, and politics all have a role in understanding change and continuity, but ideas are essential for research and innovation. In fact, the emerging powers are more directly involved in crucial normative debates about faster growth and poverty reduction. How international peace initiatives may and should be implemented, and how relevant international institutions, both individually and through new alliances like the BRICS (Brazil, Russia, India, China, and South Africa) can and should contribute to a more just system. Academics, intellectuals, and epistemic communities from all over the world may be tasked with defining the future world system we want and need in that case. Collaborations and discussions in the realm of research take place in a variety of ways. On the other hand, the global effort to rebuild multilateralism must become more comprehensive and inclusive. It must also avoid politicizing major issues, as this has inhibited government participation and, more recently, discourse (Carayannis & Weiss, 2021).

The World Bank's (2020), Governance Global Practice's (GGP) role is to enable a successful response to COVID-19 by providing a flow of infrastructure development projects to help the nations navigate heightened fragility. But we understand that resource constraints are severe, and large-scale service delivery requirements are constantly changing. The pandemic has demonstrated the significance of a stronger, flexible, and responsive public service that can mitigate risk, and respond to emergencies. It is vital to obtain life-saving treatments and supplies on an emergency basis to decrease the impact of COVID-19. Beyond COVID-19, the GGP aids the countries in establishing capable, open, efficient, inclusive, responsible, and accountable institutions. The effectiveness of the COVID-19 vaccination campaign is contingent on a large number of people receiving the vaccine quickly, equitably, and efficiently. Importantly, both the population's trust in and willingness to participate and the programme's well-functioning and government management are critical.

Governments are gearing up to rapidly deal with the COVID-19 epidemic. In this effort, according to the OECD (2021) they face three extraordinary challenges: (1) a community health crisis involving the Virus, such as diagnosing and treating infected communities; (2) widespread food and livelihood insecurity as a result of the forced halt in business and the resulting disruption in the food supply and (3) presidential action to resolve the crises and maintain public safety. Dishonesty risks jeopardizing the government's ability to respond effectively to all of these challenges, which are amplified by the magnitude and speed of the disaster.

Organization of the Book

Organization is expected in any book. A book structure or organization provides readers with clear guidelines for how to proceed and what to expect from the book ahead. This also connects readers and the authors. Chapter 2 discusses the pandemic and some conceptual issues that explain the current trying times. According to proponents of globalization theory, the world has become "one-world," or one global village. This means that the entire planet had evolved into a global community (Dixon, 2009). The inference is that something that happens in one part of the world travels quickly to the rest of the world. As global concerns, crises, and difficulties occurred, requiring international cooperation and nations cooperating in a culture of "complex interdependence," international relations were elevated to the level of global politics. The COVID-19 epidemic has created unprecedented global health, humanitarian, societal, and human rights challenges. The origins and evolution of this Coronavirus and certain theoretical intricacies are examined in this chapter. Global governance and international development cooperation, political tensions between nations, immigration, public health, prejudice, the economy, gender vulnerability, educational access, political involvement, and citizen trust are all considered.

Chapter 3 delves into politics around the pandemic, its outcomes, and its ramifications. COVID-19 is a shock to the world system, altering global politics and igniting new conflicts between friends and foes. It will have long-term geopolitical ramifications. Difficulties have beset international politics. The divide between public and private goods was widening, and multilateralism was being called into doubt. The COVID-19 pandemic, on the other hand, has accelerated these alterations while also providing a fresh opportunity to recreate the global pattern. In general, the prognosis is dismal. However, the pandemic's impact may have some silver linings. Civil society organizations working on the epidemic's front lines may be able to contribute to the community's democratic vitality. In some cases, effective state actions may be able to help restore trust in governmental or technocratic capacities. Under the current system, global governance will become more challenging to manage; nevertheless, no major institutional reform will be agreed upon and implemented anytime soon. Following on from the preceding chapter's theoretical focus, this chapter examines the political predicaments the world is and will be undergoing.

Chapter 4 focuses on post-COVID optimism and its possible ramifications. In light of COVID-19's potential to exacerbate territorial inequalities, a place-based strategy to regional development is needed that is more inclusive and urgent, as well as a renewed feeling of urgency. The importance of top-down and bottom-up activity balance, the necessity for successful connections and trust across several sets of actors, the requirement for adaptability and flexibility all contribute to this sense of urgency.

It has also reignited policy debates on regional resilience. As a result of the epidemic's demands on all levels of government, local development priorities have shifted in favour of regional resilience development. To address the issue, academics, policymakers and practitioners should avoid local-to-global collaborations and

Organization of the Book 17

instead devise practical strategies for persons whose rights are most directly affected to advance their concerns. Electoral innovation, healthcare development, educational access, and economics are the measures explored in this chapter. Chapter 4 looks at how public engagement and freedom of expression can help reduce stigma and raise awareness, improve women's financial stability, citizen trust, interconnection, helpful attitudes, and the future of globalization.

Conclusions

The COVID-19 outbreak has pushed world politics to unprecedented heights. Global and domestic political scenarios have changed. Global politics seems to have been deeply divided, and domestic politics for many countries have shifted from democracy to the revival of autocracy. The COVID-19 outbreak is the most serious threat to world order since World War II, and it threatens to undermine an already fragile international system. It has also created secondary shocks, which might destabilize the global order even more. The rules-based international system, which had brought decades of peace, prosperity, and freedom, has fallen at risk since the COVID-19 outbreak. Threats from major revisionist powers, as well as resistance within democracies, place pressure on the system. These threats continue to exist, but the pandemic has thrown a strategic curveball. The global economy is in free fall, the US-China rivalry has intensified, the transatlantic alliance has deteriorated, and seemingly helpless international institutions are facing a credibility crisis. The international order's future could go in a number of directions, ranging from a complete breakdown of the law-based global system to its revival and adaption for the twenty-first century (Cimmino et al., 2020).

COVID-19 has changed the course of history and has infiltrated every aspect of life. It also makes individuals more aware of how their lives are interwoven with the lives of others throughout the world, from financial well-being to health and sanitation. The harmful impact of COVID-19 on world health and economies currently transcends all other concerns. Yemen, Syria, and other war-torn countries are rarely covered in the mainstream media. Moreover, as well, migration does not make the front pages anymore. A new dualism has formed in the world, which some refer to as a trade-off.

Even though freedom and security are linked, the balance between supporting health and the economy has shifted the debate. Even if the epidemic is contained, it will be unevenly contained, with control ranging from country to country. This discrepancy could hurt the national economy by making countries that have successfully contained the Virus hesitant to open their borders (Yenel, 2020).

The crisis has highlighted our reliance on domestic and international mobility and the importance of foreign workers in a variety of industries, including health and agriculture. As a result, it is critical to ensure that international migration restrictions are consistently lowered and that international mobility mechanisms are sustained because of shifting labour markets, new stock and value chains, digitization, automation, and shifting work and workplace modalities. To aid in the pandemic recovery, migrant workers must be reskilled and upskilled. More effective multi-stakeholder cooperation is essential along existing and future corridors and economic sectors.

Migrants and displaced persons must be included in rehabilitation programmes, and their capacities must be reinforced in order to support long-term socio-economic growth. COVID-19 also emphasized the importance of data in assisting governments, health actors, and other stakeholders in avoiding the disease's spread. Without timely and trustworthy data, which is critical for identifying the most vulnerable communities, a comprehensive, coordinated, and successful response is impossible to deliver (IOM, 2021). The post-COVID-19 period appears to be full of shocks, demonstrating that life is again full of profound unpredictability, as the COVID-19 epidemic shook the world. With this insight, the most sensible approach to global governance is prudence. We may one day realize that the precautionary principle was the most critical moral acquired from COVID-19 if our frontrunners learn to use it to drive policy.

References

Acemoglu, D. (2010). Institutions, factor prices, and taxation: Virtues of strong states? *American Economic Review, 100*(2), 115–119.

Acemoglu, D., & Robinson, J. A. (2012). *Economic origins of dictatorship and democracy.* Cambridge University Press.

Akon, M. S., & Rahman, M. (2020). Reshaping the global order in the post covid-19 era: A critical analysis. *Chinese Journal of International Review, 2*(1), 2050006.

Alvarez, F. E., Argente, D., & Lippi, F. (2020). *A simple planning problem for Covid-19 lockdown* (No. w26981). National Bureau of Economic Research.

Ashford, E., & Kroenig, M. (2020, July 31). Is this the beginning of a new cold war with China? *Foreign Policy.* Retrieved on August 7, 2020, from https://foreignpolicy.com/2020/07/31/is-this-the-beginning-of-a-new-cold-war-with-china/

Bartels, L. M. (2008). *Unequal democracy: The political economy of the new gilded age.* Princeton University Press.

Beirne, J., Morgan, P. J., & Sonobe, T. (Eds.). (2021). *Introduction: COVID-19 impacts and policy options: An Asian perspective* (pp. 1–10). Asian Development Bank.

Benton, J. E. (2018). Intergovernmental relations in the earlier twenty-first century: Lingering images of further phases and emergence of a new phase. In C. W. Stenberg & D. K. Hamilton (Eds.), *Intergovernmental relations in transition: Reflections and directions* (pp. 15–36). Routledge.

Beramendi, P., & Christopher, J. A. (Eds.). (2008). *Democracy, inequality, and representation: A comparative perspective.* Russell Sage Foundation.

Bowman, A. O. M., & Kearney, R. C. (2007). The resurgent states in the intergovernmental system: Cooperation and conflict. In G. R. Stephens & N. Wikstrom (Eds.), *American intergovernmental relations: A fragmented federal polity* (pp. 159–187). Oxford University Press.

Brown, F. Z., Brechenmacher, S., & Carothers, T. (2020, April 6). How will the Coronavirus reshape democracy and governance globally? *Carnegie Endowment for International Peace.* https://carnegieendowment.org/2020/04/06/how-will-coronavirus-reshape-democracy-and-governance-globally-pub-81470. Accessed 30 July 2021.

References

Bump, P. (2022, February 2). *Americans have lost 13.5 million years of life during the pandemic.* https://www.washingtonpost.com/politics/2022/02/02/americans-have-lost-135-million-years-life-during-pandemic/. Accessed 28 Feb 2022.

Burke, B. F., & Brudney, J. L. (2018). Why we fight. In C. W. Stenberg & D. K. Hamilton (Eds.), *Intergovernmental relations in transition* (pp. 58–74). Routledge.

Byrne, J. P. (2012). *Encyclopedia of the black death.* ABC CLIO.

Carayannis, T., & Weiss, T. G. (2021). The 'Third' UN: Imagining post-COVID-19 multilateralism. *Global Policy, 12*(1), 5–14.

Cimmino, J., Katz, R., Kroenig, M., Lipsky, J., & Pavel, B. (2020). *A global strategy for shaping the post-COVID-19 world.* The Atlantic Council of the United States.

De Mauro, A., Greco, M., & Grimaldi, M. (2016). A formal definition of Big Data based on its essential features. *Library Review, 65*(3), 122–135.

Dixon, V. K. (2009). Understanding the implications of a global village. *Inquiries Journal, 1*(11). http://www.inquiriesjournal.com/articles/1681/understanding-the-implications-of-a-global-village

Donthu, N., & Gustafsson, A. (2020). Effects of COVID-19 on business and research. *Journal of Business Research, 117*, 284–289.

Doran, M. (2020). *How will the world look after the Covid-19 crisis?* http://sam.gov.tr/pdf/sam-yayinlari/The%20World%20after%20COVID19.pdf. Accessed 30 July 2021.

Economist. (2021, January 9). *What is the economic cost of covid-19?* https://www.economist.com/finance-and-economics/2021/01/09/what-is-the-economic-cost-of-covid-19. Accessed 7 Aug 2020.

Eiran, E. (2020). *COVID-19 and great power rivalry.* http://sam.gov.tr/pdf/sam-yayinlari/The%20World%20after%20COVID19.pdf. Accessed 30 July 2021.

Enderwick, P., & Buckley, P. J. (2020). Rising regionalization: Will the post-COVID-19 world see a retreat from globalization? *Transnational Corporations Journal, 27*(2), 99–112.

Fazio, R. H., Ruisch, B. C., Moore, C. A., Granados Samayoa, J. A., Boggs, S. T., & Ladanyi, J. T. (2021). Who is (not) complying with the US social distancing directive and why? Testing a general framework of compliance with virtual measures of social distancing. *PloS one, 16*(2), e0247520.

Feng, Q. (2021, May 6). China and India can cooperate on COVID-19 fight but tensions still in air. *Global Times.* https://www.globaltimes.cn/page/202105/1222812.shtml

Ferdous, J., & Ullah, A. K. M. A. (2022). COVID-19 and migrant population in South Asia: Exploring the resilience. *IJAPS, 18*(2).

Freedom House. (2020, October 2). Democracy under lockdown—The impact of COVID-19 on. *Global Freedom.* https://freedomhouse.org/article/new-report-democracy-under-lockdown-impact-covid-19-global-freedom. Accessed 16 May 2021.

Gale, J. (2021, November 8). *COVID stole 28 million years of life from 31 countries last year.* https://www.bloomberg.com/news/articles/2021-11-09/covid-stole-28-million-years-of-life-from-31-countries-last-year. Accessed 19 May 2021.

Global Times. (2021, July 20). 55 countries submit joint letters to WHO, opposing politicization of COVID-19 origins study. *Global Times.* https://www.globaltimes.cn/page/202107/1229118.shtml. Accessed 1 Aug 2021.

Goodman, C. B., Hatch, M. E., & McDonald, B. D., III. (2021). State preemption of local laws: Origins and modern trends. *Perspectives on Public Management and Governance, 4*(2), 146–158.

Gottfried, A. E. (1983). Intrinsic motivation in young children. *Young Children, 39*(1), 64–73.

Greer, S., King, E., Fonseca, E., & Peralta-Santos, A. (Eds.). (2021). *Coronavirus politics: The comparative politics and policy of COVID-19.* University of Michigan Press. https://doi.org/10.3998/mpub.11927713

Hall, C. M., & Prayag, G. (2020). Earthquakes and tourism: Impacts, responses and resilience – An introduction. In C. M. Hall & G. Prayag (Eds.), *Tourism and earthquakes.* Channel View.

Hall, J., Gaved, M., & Sargent, J. (2021). Participatory research approaches in times of Covid-19: A narrative literature review. *International Journal of Qualitative Methods, 20*, 16094069211010088.

Hays, J. N. (2005). *Epidemics and pandemics: Their impacts on human history*. ABC-CLIO.

International Centre for Not-for-profit Law (ICNPL). (2021, August 1). *COVID-19 civic freedom tracker*. https://www.icnl.org/covid19tracker/?issue=5. Accessed 9 Feb 2021.

International Institute for Strategic Studies (IISS). (2020). IISS Manama dialogue 2020 special publication: The strategic and geo-economic Implications of the COVID-19 Pandemic. *The International Institute for Strategic Studies*. https://www.iiss.org/blogs/research-paper/2020/12/strategic-geo-economic-implications-covid-19-pandemic. Accessed 30 July 2021.

International Organization for Migration (IOM). (2021). *IOM strategic response and recovery plan COVID-19*. International Organization for Migration.

Jeff, L.-S. (2021). *COVID-19 updates: Helping employers navigate workplace challenges*. https://www.wtwco.com/en-US/Insights/campaigns/covid-19-updates-helping-employers-navigate-workplace-challenges

Jeong, A. (2021). *A study of 37 nations estimates the extra years lost in 2020 total 28 million and found a greater decline in life expectancy among males*. https://www.washingtonpost.com/health/2021/11/04/coronavirus-pandemic-global-years-lost-life/. Accessed 3 July 2021.

Kahf, A. (2020). *The "new normal" global governance post COVID-19*. http://sam.gov.tr/pdf/sam-yayinlari/The%20World%20after%20COVID19.pdf. Accessed 30 July 2021.

Karabell, Z. (2020). *Will the Coronavirus bring the end of globalization? Don't count on it*. https://www.wsj.com/articles/will-the-coronavirus-bring-the-end-of-globalization-dont-count-on-it-11584716305. Accessed 21 July 2021.

Liu, Y. (2020, December 07). *COVID-19 & war? Do India and China only have two choices?* Observer Research Foundation. https://www.orfonline.org/expert-speak/covid19-war-do-india-and-china-only-have-two-choices/. Accessed 1 July 2021.

Luscombe, R. (2020, March 23). Cuomo wins praise for "wisdom" amid coronavirus crisis as Trump blusters. *The Guardian*. https://www.theguardian.com/world/2020/mar/23/cuomo-wins-praise-for-wisdom-amid-coronavirus-crisis-as-trump-blusters. Accessed 1 June 2021.

Maestre, J. M. (2020). *Finis Coronabit Virvs*. http://selat.org/data/documents/00_FINIS_CORONA BIT_VIRVS_JoseMariaMaestreMaestre_SELat.pdf. Accessed 15 May 2020.

Ministry of Foreign Affairs, the People's Republic of China. (2021). *Do not let the political virus contaminate the origin-tracing of COVID-19*. https://www.fmprc.gov.cn/mfa_eng/wjb_663304/zwjg_665342/zwbd_665378/t1900315.shtml. Accessed 17 May 2021.

Mohan, D. (2020). *A broad crisis of public distrust that we need to resolve*. http://dspace.jgu.edu.in:8080/jspui/bitstream/10739/4281/1/A%20broad%20crisis%20of%20public%20distrust%20.pdf. Accessed 30 July 2021.

Mueller, D. C. (2003). *Public choice III*. Cambridge University Press.

Muurlink, O. T., & Taylor-Robinson, A. W. (2020). COVID-19: Cultural predictors of gender differences in global prevalence patterns. *Frontiers in Public Health, 8*, 174. https://doi.org/10.3389/fpubh.2020.00174/full

Noury, A., François, A., Gergaud, O., & Garel, A. (2021). How does COVID-19 affect electoral participation? Evidence from the French municipal elections. *PloS one, 16*(2), e0247026.

OECD. (2021). *The territorial impact of COVID-19: Managing the crisis and recovery across levels of government*. https://www.oecd.org/coronavirus/policy-responses/the-territorial-impact-of-covid-19-managing-the-crisis-and-recovery-across-levels-of-government-a2c6abaf/. Accessed 7 Mar 2021.

Pal, P. (2020, June 20). Managing a post-COVID global order: Looking through the lens of international relations: Extraordinary and plenipotentiary. *Diplomatist*. https://diplomatist.com/2020/06/20/managing-a-post-covid-global-order-looking-through-the-lens-of-international-relations/. Accessed 4 Aug 2021.

Perthes, V. (2020, March 31). *The Corona crisis and international relations: Open questions, tentative assumptions*. German Institute for International and Security Affairs. https://www.

References

swp-berlin.org/en/publication/the-corona-crisis-and-international-relations-open-questions-ten tative-assumptions. Accessed 30 July 2021.

Piccarozzi, M., Silvestri, C., & Morganti, P. (2021). COVID-19 in management studies: A systematic literature review. *Sustainability, 13*(7), 3791.

Piketty, T. (2014). *Capital in the twenty-first century.* Harvard University Press.

Powell, K. (2012). Facing anti-vaccine movements: Myths and facts about adverse events. *International Journal of Infectious Diseases, 16*, e57–e58.

Rahman, M. K., Gazi, M. A. I., Bhuiyan, M. A., & Rahaman, M. A. (2021). Effect of Covid-19 pandemic on tourist travel risk and management perceptions. *PLoS ONE, 16*(9), e0256486. https://doi.org/10.1371/journal.pone.0256486

Ranger, T., & Slack, P. (Eds.). (1992). *Epidemics and ideas: Essays on the historical perception of pestilence.* Cambridge University Press.

Repucci, S., & Slipowitz, A. (2020). The impact of COVID-19 on the global struggle for freedom. *Freedom House.* https://freedomhouse.org/report/special-report/2020/democracy-under-lockdown. Accessed 12 Feb 2021.

Ritzen, Y. (2021, March 8). Bangladesh bought phone-hacking tools from Israel. *Aljazeera.* https://www.aljazeera.com/news/2021/3/8/bangladesh-bought-hacking-tools-from-isr ael-documents-show. Accessed 16 Feb 2021.

Sassanelli, C., Rosa, P., Rocca, R., & Terzi, S. (2019). Circular economy performance assessment methods: A systematic literature review. *Journal of Cleaner Production, 229*, 440–453.

Sawada, Y., & Sumulong, L. R. (2021). Macroeconomic impacts of the COVID-19 pandemic in developing Asia. In J. Beirne, P. J. Morgan, & T. Sonobe (Eds.), *COVID-19 impacts and policy options: An Asian perspective* (pp. 11–47). Asian Development Bank.

Snowden, F. M. (2020). *Epidemics and society: From the black death to the present.* Yale University Press.

Torreblanca, J. I. (2020). *The impact of COVID-19.* http://sam.gov.tr/pdf/sam-yayinlari/The%20W orld%20after%20COVID19.pdf. Accessed 30 July 2021.

Trent, J., & Schnurr, L. (2018). *A United Nations renaissance: What the UN is, and what it could be.* Verlag Barbara Budrich. https://doi.org/10.3224/84740711

Turner, J. (2020, April 15). 'Starved for content': Ron DeSantis explains why sporting events are needed now. *Tampa Bay Times.* https://www.tampabay.com/news/health/2020/04/14/in-defense-of-wwe-decision-ron-desantis-said-he-wants-more-sporting-events/. Accessed 19 Sept 2021.

Ullah, A. A., Hossain, M. A., & Huque, A. S. (2021). Non-conventional migration: An evolving pattern in South Asia. *Journal of African and Asian Studies, 56*(3), 00219096211008468.

Ullah, A. K. M. A., & Azizuddin, M. (2018). South Asian student migration to Nordic countries: Changing initial motivations. *Asian Profile, 46*(1), 73–87.

Ulutaş, U. (2020). *The World after COVID-19: Cooperation or competition?* Center for Strategic Research (SAM), Turkish Ministry of Foreign Affairs.

Vos, R., Martin W., & Laborde, D. (2020, March 20). How much will global poverty increase because of COVID-19? *IFPRI.* https://www.ifpri.org/blog/how-much-will-global-poverty-increase-bec ause-covid-19. Accessed 29 Aug 2021.

Warner-Mackintosh, I. (2020, November 26). *Covid-19: Participatory action research as emergency response.* Centre for Culture, Sport and Events (CCSE) Blog. http://ccse.uws.ac.uk/2020/11/26/ covid-19-participatory-action-research-as-emergency-response/. Accessed 30 July 2021.

Williams, B. (2020). The politics of a pandemic. *Political Insight, 11*(3), 37–39.

Wintermeyer, L. (2020). *Covid and the new world order—Building A new human centered economy.* https://www.forbes.com/sites/lawrencewintermeyer/2020/09/17/coivd-and-the-new-world-orderbuiding-a-new-human-centered-economy/?sh=c67c6678f0c3. Accessed 23 Oct 2021.

Wired. (2020). *Zoom took over the world: This is what will happen next.* https://www.wired.co.uk/ article/future-of-zoom. Accessed 28 Feb 2022.

World Bank. (2020). *Monitoring COVID-19 impacts on households in Mongolia.* https://www.worldbank.org/en/country/mongolia/brief/monitoring-covid-19-impacts-on-households-in-mongolia. Accessed 1 Aug 2021.

Yenel, S. (2020). *The effects of COVID-19 and how to prepare for the future: Challenges of global governance amid the COVID-19 pandemic.* Council on Foreign Relations: International Institutions and Global Governance Program.

Zhou, X., Snoswell, C. L., Harding, L. E., Bambling, M., Edirippulige, S., Bai, X., & Smith, A. C. (2020, April). The role of Telehealth in reducing the mental health burden from COVID-19. *Telemedicine and e-Health, 26*(4), 377–379. https://doi.org/10.1089/tmj.2020.0068

Chapter 2
Underlying Conceptual Approach:
An Era or a Crisis?

Introduction

In the previous chapter, we established the research questions, the aims, the argument we intended to make, and the structure of the book. We linked to emphasize the critical nature of the research we conducted during the pandemic, as well as the ways in which global politics are evolving in reaction to the pandemic and vaccine politics. As a result of the disputes ignited in the preceding chapter, the book requires a firm theoretical foundation about previous pandemics, politics, and the path to resolution. The objective of this chapter is to tie it to the remainder of the book's argument. This chapter examines some prominent theories that attempt to explain the crisis, pandemics, and crisis-related global politics. We address how we intend to convey the preceding chapter's objective. We begin by defining crisis and pandemic. Then, we outline our research methodology. We briefly outline the research approaches we used.

We conducted a thorough literature search to ascertain how previous scientists defined and connected these fundamental concepts to the pandemics. After analyzing numerous models and theories, we arrived at the definitions that best fit our research and explained why. The theoretical framework is critical because it acts as the lens through which our research challenges and questions will be seen. Explaining the theories enables us to demonstrate why the theory we chose is appropriate for use in the book and to demonstrate how the theory relates to our investigation.

This chapter covers the literature on the application of theories in pandemic and emergency response situations in order to inform pandemic modeling, research, and public health practice. Pandemics have had a profound impact on human history, destroying empires, reshaping colonization patterns, and giving people advantages in the marketplace. Depending on the circumstances, it can also rearrange labour markets, potentially far-reaching repercussions for inequality and social organization. Indeed, if a pandemic creates a large enough population shock, it has the potential to drastically alter labour and capital's relative bargaining power. This raises the

---

© The Author(s), under exclusive license to Springer Nature Singapore Pte Ltd. 2022   23
AKM. A. Ullah and J. Ferdous, *The Post-Pandemic World and Global Politics*,
https://doi.org/10.1007/978-981-19-1910-7_2

prospect of pandemics having long-term consequences for the content and behaviour of politics (Gingerich & Vogler, 2021).

Globalization introduced the concept of "one-worldness," or viewing the world as a single space connected in real-time through improved communication and information technologies. The entire planet had effectively become a global community (McLuhan & Moos, 2014). "One-worldness" is considered a great thing. However, it has some downsides. As one problem starts one corner of the world, it spreads fast to the other corner. As global problems, crises, and difficulties arose, international relations became important to global politics, requiring international cooperation, states working together in a culture of "complex interdependence" Environmental challenges, gender issues, civil rights, world markets, and violent extremism have all emerged as global issues that may play a role in defining global security (Pal, 2020; Ullah et al., 2020). The COVID-19 epidemic has engendered global health, humanitarian, socioeconomic, and human rights crisis that has never been seen before. While the number of cases and deaths worldwide continues to rise, the containment measures put in place to stop COVID-19 from spreading—such as travel restrictions—have revealed the enormous human and economic consequences, particularly for those on the move.

While immunization efforts are underway, many public health systems are overburdened and unable to cope with the crisis's size and scope. Barriers to accessing essential services, such as COVID-19 vaccines, persist in many nations for migrants, displaced populations, and other vulnerable groups (IOM, 2021). On top of the fact that the COVID-19 outbreak has claimed millions of lives around the world, it poses a global threat to human health and food security to that scale that the world has never seen before. As time passes by, we see the pandemic has caused havoc on the society and economy, leaving millions of people on the verge of starvation. The outbreak has affected the entire food supply chain, exposing its susceptibility. Farmers and farm workers were unable to exchange goods because of restrictions and confinement measures, which disrupted local and international food chains and limited access to food and safety. Millions of lives have been put in jeopardy as a result of the pandemic (WHO, 2020a).

The pandemic has implications on democracy, government, public health, and the global economy. COVID arrived when democracy was under fire in many parts of the world, and it risks exacerbating democratic retrenchment and autocratic consolidation. Several governments have already used the pandemic to enhance executive power and curtail individual liberty. However, such acts are simply the tip of the iceberg in some countries (Brown et al., 2020).

The highly contagious nature of SARS-CoV-2 necessitated lockdowns as a quick response to impose social distancing norms and prevent aggressive transmission. Schools, workplaces, public transportation, and recreational spaces such as retail malls, movie theatres, hotels, and restaurants were closed, implying that every walk of life to some extent was impacted. Domestic violence increased, mental health conditions worsened, healthcare systems were overburdened, and income and financial health were ruined. All crises disproportionately impact marginalized populations, and early assessments from civil society groups, research organizations, and even

Introduction   25

the media reveal that the crisis negatively impacts residents. The epidemic has the potential to undo decades of progress accomplished (Lewis, 2020). Many women's livelihoods have been directly harmed by the lockdowns and closures, which could ruin years of financial success (Ullah et al., 2021). It had an impact on corporate operations, causing millions of migrant workers to lose their employment. All sorts of violence, exploitation, and abuse increase instability, poverty, marginalization, and the disintegration of social cohesiveness. Because survivors are trapped with their abusers owing to travel restrictions, the epidemic has increased the suscepti-bility of girls and women to gender-based violence (GBV) all over the world. It has heightened the risks of extortion and trafficking as well.

While the COVID-19 virus is essentially a health crisis, it has worsened the existing vulnerabilities, created extensive economic disruptions, and resulted in a slew of additional humanitarian and protection requirements. Those in unstable, disaster-prone, and conflict-affected countries—including frontline relief workers—face major risks as community propagation and socioeconomic consequences persist, worsened by limits in the supply of life-saving humanist assistance. Simultane-ously, crisis-affected individuals, particularly those homeless and living in communal settings, frequently reside in highly populated places with already overburdened health systems, no resources to control and prevent infection, and unequal access to essential services.

As a result, the COVID-19 epidemic has drastically heightened protection concerns, particularly in vulnerable settings. COVID-19 has enhanced the vulner-ability of migrants and displaced communities, and had profound socioeconomic implications due to reducing national and international mobility, affecting trade corridors, supply chains, and labour markets and creating a major worldwide reces-sion. Unemployment, insecurity, and inequalities are now on the rise, with knock-on impacts on severe poverty, food insecurity, and livelihoods, hitting individuals on the move in particular. Seasonal migrant worker programmes in many countries have been halted. The tourism sector has come to a halt, putting many countries and city-states, particularly in the global South, out of business.

Furthermore, the imposition of border restrictions and travel embargos have left many travellers and migrants stranded, including seasonal labourers, temporary resi-dents, international students, tourists, mariners, and others (Ullah et al., 2021). The vulnerable communities' support has been disrupted, resulting in increased security concerns and the need for assistance. The epidemic has also exacerbated discrim-ination and prejudice against migrants. Extended lockdown measures increased the likelihood of xenophobia, which is worsened by social tensions caused by the economic slump. The government shutdown has compounded the precarious situa-tion the migrant people are already in since they face unemployment, and millions of migrant workers are finding it extremely hard to return to their country. Migrants and other disadvantaged groups are frequently affected on two fronts: in their destination countries and their families in their home countries. The families that are dependent on remittances in low—and—middle countries will be deeply shocked. Compared to pre-COVID-19 in 2019, the remittance is predicted to shrink by 14% in 2021 as the COVID-19 outbreak and economic crisis develop (World Bank, 2020), and we assume that the declining trend will continue to stay a few more years until the world comes back to normal, if at all.

The Global South is faced with a difficult paradox: bringing food to the table and maintaining social distance (i.e. maintaining social distance and isolation and work daily and obtain bread is practically conflicting). Significant reductions in livelihood prospects have worsened community tensions and curtailed opportunities for economic generation and self-sufficiency in fragile situations (IOM, 2021).

In the immediate aftermath of the pandemic's discovery, the public was inundated with fear-inducing information. Since the outbreak scientists and journalists have been working relentlessly to determine how COVID-19 spreads, how fast and its impact. Political leaders used a range of strategies to promote their own opinions and public health objectives. In the United States, political leaders on both sides of the aisle enthusiastically seized the intelligence and steered their respective parties in the right direction. Significant disparities existed in how people received scientific facts and responded to safety concerns, which had an effect on the rate of virus propagation (Mana et al., 2021).

Hardy et al. (2021) found that voters on the left were distrustful of former US President Trump, political leaders, and large corporations. The left demonstrated a greater level of faith in scientists. Before and during the outbreak, interviews and surveys highlighted economic inequality and capitalism as contributing causes of the public health disaster. Outliers on the extreme left joked about being "cooked like frogs in a carefully heated pot." They were also more likely to report hate crimes and public attacks during the pandemic.

The pandemic has halted many industries to kick off their production, and hence it delayed foreign recruitment; besides, in most developing countries, the internal business has nearly ceased. Without a comprehensive, selfless, economic stimulus plan coordinated by powerful countries, the suffering of the laid-off and unemployed workers may grow by the day. Many countries in the developing world cannot replicate the safeguard measures taken by their wealthier peers and are relying on hot weather to keep the disease at bay. Countries in the Global South are feeling the most severe financial consequences. Poor public health monitoring equipment, poverty, and backwardness (in many forms) are all disadvantages that cannot be overcome by a favourable environment (Pal, 2020).

This magnitude of the consequences of the pandemic necessitates an explanation of comparable significance (Leman & Cinnirella, 2007) for psychological advantage such as it provides a sense of control. Conspiracy theories have long been associated with a lack of control, which makes sense given this rationale. Even though these patterns are false, people use them to compensate for their lack of control in the real world (e.g., Douglas et al., 2017). This pandemic is a perfect breeding ground for conspiracy theories since there is no obvious mechanical explanation for the illness, which interrupts people's lives and leaves them in a condition of confusion (Van Bavel et al., 2020). Although this general pattern appears to be one of the most robust conclusions in conspiracy theory, in the current COVID-19 situation, two popular conspiracy theories appeared to be theoretically incompatible and associated with divergent behaviours. While many people downplayed the threat of COVID-19, comparing it to the flu, and suspected others of making false claims for their gain (e.g., harming national economies, passing unpopular/restrictive laws), others painted a more bleak picture, claiming that the new coronavirus had not evolved by mutation but had been purposefully manufactured and spread as a bioweapon for political or economic gain (Andersen et al., 2020).

Experts say this is not a new phenomenon, according to past research, believing in conspiracy surges during pandemics (e.g., Van Prooijen & Douglas, 2017). Every significant incident has been met with a slew of conspiracy theories alleging that influential operatives orchestrated covert schemes in the last few decades. For example, The Soviet Committee for State Security (Geissler & Sprinkle, 2013) depicted HIV/AIDS as a biological weapon, and the prevalent idea that AIDS is a plot to destroy black people has a direct impact on preventative behaviour (Geissler & Sprinkle, 2013), for example, use of condoms or pre-exposure prophylaxis (Bogart & Thorburn, 2005; Bogart et al., 2010). During the 2015 and 2016 Zika outbreaks, rumours circulated that the virus spread due to genetically modified mosquitos or that governments employed the virus to intentionally kill people (see Klofstad et al., 2019). An equally important explanation is needed for such incidents (Leman & Cinnirella, 2007).

Explanations have a number of psychological advantages, one of which is that they help people feel more in control of their lives. Conspiracy theories have been linked to a lack of control, which is not surprising. Individuals who are unable to control their surroundings resort to recognizing patterns, even if they are entirely fake (e.g., Douglas et al., 2017). There is no readily available mechanical explanation for the present coronavirus epidemic, which disrupts people's lives and leaves them in a state of chaos (Imhoff & Lamberty, 2020; Van Bavel et al., 2020).

Conspiracy theories as well may have a positive side effect of giving people a sense of control. Even while these conspiracy theories highlight valid concerns, we believe they may lead to inappropriate behaviour in the current context (Imhoff & Bruder, 2014). Several specialists have been among the most outspoken advocates for "flattening the curve" and reducing infection transmission during this coronavirus outbreak. Confusion mentality, defined as the popular notion that great forces conspire to govern the world, has been connected to mistrust in science in general, and in the biomedical system in particular, due to its perceived authority (Galliford & Furnham, 2017; Lamberty & Imhoff, 2018; Oliver & Wood, 2014). People who believe in conspiracy theories are especially hesitant to heed professional advice on how to limit the number of people who become ill.

A person's risk assessment is directly influenced by their perception of illness-related dangers, and this impression determines health-promoting self-care behaviours (Ferrer & Klein, 2015). A stronger sense of danger, for example, is linked to a more protective response. COVID-19 is being misreported or a hoax, and people are less likely to comply with official suggestions like handwashing and social isolation and distance if they believe the government is exaggerating the situation (Stanley et al., 2020). We think that downplaying the consequence of the pandemic undermines the people who died of COVID-19.

Coronavirus skepticism spans the political spectrum, with conservative and progressive political ideologies adherent. While some left-wing civil libertarians opposed to the lockdowns questioned the virus's severity, the political right-wing has been the most vocal in their opposition. The global response to the pandemic has mirrored the attitudes of some fringe political parties, who regard it as an infringement on their individual liberties. Right-wing groups, for example, view the coronavirus in this way because they believe everything is a government conspiracy. It would be "government seeking illegitimately to close enterprises, kill jobs, and limit how close people can stand to one another (Slessor, 2020).

As the COVID-19 epidemic rose worldwide, it elicited unprecedented policy reactions and threw major societal institutions into disarray—from work policy and business networks to individual/family interaction styles. While the pandemic's evolution is uncertain, its appearance in the first half of 2020 raised concerns about its position as a public health emergency, a global downturn, and a blaster of central governance institutions (Cotula, 2021). Most of the countries affected went into statewide lockdown to keep the virus's transmission minimum. Due to the government's clout, the situation improved steadily in China, but it deteriorated in many other regions. United Kingdom (UK), Italy, France, Spain, Germany, and other European countries were among the worst affected. With the most considerable number of total cases and deaths, the United States is experiencing the worst problem as a single country (Akon & Rahman, 2020).

The Origin Theory Discourse

SARS and MERS were initially associated with COVID-19's emergence, but it has subsequently been shown to have far more devastating consequences. About 40 million people died from influenza during the 1918–1920 pandemic (Barro et al., 2020). When extrapolated to today's global population, this equates to approximately 150 million deaths. COVID-19 deaths are unlikely to reach the magnitude of those during the influenza pandemic of 1918, given the progress in public health since then and the use of pharmaceutical and non-pharmaceutical measures to restrict the spread of COVID-19 (Sawada & Sumulong, 2021). Anthrax from the Middle East or SARS have pulversied economies around the world in the recent past. At least 26 economies were affected by SARS in 2003; these included Hong Kong and China, Singapore, Taiwan and Viet Nam. Malaysia, the Philippines, South Korea, and Thailand were among the countries where MERS quickly spread after it was detected in Saudi Arabia in 2012 (Shinozaki & Rao, 2021).

The origins and evolution of this coronavirus (COVID-19) may be traced back to the Chinese province of Hubei, in which the first cases were detected in December 2019 (Zhang et al., 2020). The case number was climbing rapidly and spread horizontally to sweep the entire world, and hence the World Health Organization (WHO) formally declared a global pandemic on March 11, 2020 (Wu et al., 2020). The pandemic was first detected in the United States and Western Europe, spreading disproportionately in high-traffic cities which serve as international transit hubs (Bonotti & Zech, 2021). However, that was too late, or the virus spread around the world, leading to a shortage of preparedness and prevention for most governments. The ability of states to communicate with one another was critical in spreading the virus in this scenario (Akon & Rahman, 2020).

A few possible theories explain the origins of the coronavirus pandemic that has claimed more than five million lives as of December 2021. The first possibility is the well-known zoonotic spillover pathway, in which a pathogen spreads from animal to human. The second possibility is that a laboratory in Wuhan, China, was doing dangerous research with bat coronaviruses and may have experienced an accidental leak. Neither idea is supported by evidence, but as 18 notable scientists point out, both continue to be plausible, the world must be informed (*Washington Post*, 2021). A better understanding of the origins of this pandemic is essential, according to specialists. Ralph Baric, a coronavirus expert from the University of North Carolina at Chapel Hill, was one of the 18 scientists who participated in the Wuhan Institute of Virology. Relman and Bloom organized the letter, which was endorsed by Rep. Anna Eshoo (D-Calif.), chair of the House Energy and Commerce health subcommittee, who is also a Stanford University professor. It urges for "appropriate investigation" that is "open, data-driven, inclusive of various experts, subject to independent review, and responsibly managed to minimize the impact of conflicts-of-interest," citing a prior World Health Organization-China investigation that was imbalanced (*Washington Post*, 2021).

The World Health Organization (WHO) was tasked with determining how SARS-CoV-2 transferred from animals to humans. The tasks include whether it transferred via the cold/food chain; direct zoonotic introduction; and laboratory-induced introduction all fall within the intermediate host category. Transmission to humans via intermediary host: According to WHO, the novel coronavirus is most likely to spread when an infected animal infects another animal, which then infects a human. Unbeknownst to them, the sick [infected] person transmitted the virus to anyone with whom they came into touch, resulting in a pandemic (Douglas, 2021). Although the virus has been detected in bats and pangolins, there is still no proof that it has spread from one species to another. The WHO team believes that this is because the virus may have gone through an animal intermediary before coming into contact with a person. Although highly contagious in humans, the SARS-CoV-2 virus appears to be highly versatile and can infect a wide range of animals as well (WHO, 2021).

Contamination from a previously afflicted animal: It's also possible that SARS-CoV-2 was transferred to humans via animal-to-human transmission. This hypothesis proposes that the SARS-CoV-2 virus was spread from an animal to a human by direct contact (i.e. without any animal acting as an intermediary). Person-to-person contact and super-spreading episodes aided the virus's propagation. According to this notion, bats, pangolins, and even minks have been infected with a virus remarkably similar to the SARS-CoV-2 virus (Bertin et al., 2020). The likelihood of a person coming into contact with any of the aforementioned animals may go against this notion. Farm and domestic animals are more prone to come into contact with humans.

Theory of refrigerated food: The WHO and other health professionals believe this notion to be plausible. According to this argument, frozen food products may have served as vehicles for the virus's spread from one infected animal to a large population. The virus could have transmitted through the food itself or through the container it came in contact with. The virus has been found in frozen goods imported into China, but the evidence is scant. However, there is no solid proof that SARS-CoV-2 can be transmitted through food, and the chances of a cold chain becoming contaminated with the virus from a reservoir are extremely low (Bai, 2020).

Theory of laboratory leakage: It is possible, though unlikely, that the virus was created in a lab in China or that it was accidentally leaked there. According to this idea, a lab staff member became infected by mistake, and the virus subsequently spread across the facility. Scientists have examined the virus' DNA, and the report concludes that it was not intentionally unleashed (Eban, 2021). Researchers at the Wuhan Institute of Virology, the lab at the centre of the controversy, combed through their files to see whether they found any similar viruses to the coronavirus they were accused of producing. They came up empty-handed.

In Peter Ben Embarek's words, nobody has been able to pick up any hard arguments or proof or evidence that any of these labs would have been implicated in a lab leak disaster (WHO, 2021). There is also evidence that the labs involved in researching bat coronaviruses were not interested in "well-run, with a health monitoring scheme for employees, and no one had symptoms of COVID-19. Workers who had undergone SARS-CoV-2-specific serology screening (Bai, 2020; Lewandowsky & Cook, 2020) showed no signs of infection.

The lab leak theory deserves further investigation. Not to disparage Asians or China, nor is it to promote the Trump administration's use of leak propagation to divert attention away from its problems. Due to unsolved issues concerning the research being undertaken at Wuhan Institute to modify viral genome to impart new properties on them (e.g. the ability to infect new host species or transfer more easily across hosts), the study was prompted by this fact (*Washington Post*, 2021).

Conspiracy theories are separate from other types of deception and misinformation. They are distinct methods in which we make sense of the complex and occasionally unpleasant world in which we live. Additionally, they have always been viewed as a distinctly political phenomenon. According to the American historian Richard Hofstadter, such views serve as the foundation for a "paranoid style" of political thinking characterized by "heated exaggeration, suspiciousness, and conspiratorial fantasy" (Lor et al., 2021). A more recent interpretation of their significance can be found in the work of political theorist Alfred Moore, who believes they are used to explain unjustified, improbable, or even harmful events or phenomena by evoking ever-deeper conspiracies and ignoring all contradicting evidence (Dacombe, 2021).

To ensure the group's survival and existence, the conspiracy concept should be widely shared to show the horrifying truth about the threatened community. On the New World Order agenda, globalist economic and political forces are trying to undermine the sovereignty and independence of free states, according to the COVID-19 conspiracy theories (Bieber, 2020). After a catastrophic event, secret operators acquire power and consolidate authority in ways that violate constitutionally mandated rights, freedoms, and legal protections. Conspiracy theories may range in their ultimate goals and instruments, but they are almost always geared at suppressing anti-masking views and behaviours. It contains all of the elements necessary to support the conspiracy theory: Conspiracy theories can be supported with credible and verifiable evidence; affluent and powerful persons are known participants in the conspiracies (Ball & Maxmen, 2020; Evstatieva, 2020).

It is all too easy to become ensnared in theories. Individuals are capable of concocting an infinite number of fascinating stories. At a time when public trust in governments and the news media is at an all-time low, there are plenty of conspiracy theorists eager to emerge and impose their agenda on a gullible public. The only restriction of science is that it cannot fight fire with fire. When someone argues that a virus was bioengineered, scientists are compelled to state "we did not find proof" or "the weight of evidence indicates," even if the assertion is near-100% definite. However, this is how science works. It is careful in its approach. That is also one of its drawbacks. However, to keep in mind that "when two competing theories make identical predictions, the simpler one is usually confirmed" (Medical Futurist, 2020).

The Foundation of Crisis Models

The outbreak has resulted in significant behavioural shifts in both the home and the workplace. Countries around the world have implemented a variety of public health measures, including lockdowns, isolation of those who have been exposed or sick, and contact tracing to locate others who may have been infected but have not been diagnosed. Lockdowns, uncertainty, and a lack of trust have contributed to a major slowdown in economic activity in many countries. A major economic downturn may have happened as a result of this pandemic's protracted duration and wide-ranging legislative measures. Governments worldwide have implemented a variety of economic policy measures in addition to health policy solutions to mitigate the possible economic impact of COVID-19 (Fernando & McKibbin, 2021).

COVID-19 was the subject of a wide range of public awareness campaigns, as well as efforts to improve respiratory hygiene and strengthen health systems' ability to conduct testing, contact tracing and quarantining in the absence of a vaccine. Major economies instituted travel restrictions and lockdowns until a vaccine was developed. Many governments, however, have been unwilling to establish or maintain these policies for an extended period of time because of the enormous economic consequences. Infection and death rates rose dramatically when there were no severe controls on movement or lockdowns. People were killed, and economic costs surged as countries experimented with alternative techniques in real time. As of June 2020, the world had enough information to predict the pandemic's most likely outcomes, allowing policymakers to better understand the macroeconomic effects of a prolonged epidemic (Fernando & McKibbin, 2021).

Lindemann's seminal (1953) study establishes a firm theoretical foundation for the crisis. By incorporating appropriate psycho- and sociological theories, we can widen and develop the body of knowledge, as scholars and practitioners have done. As a result, theories and practices centred on crises developed, demonstrating that the previous concentration on psychodynamic perspectives was insufficient. We concur with James and Gilliland (2017) when they state that the appropriate balance of developmental, social, psychosomatic, ecological, and environmental factors should be considered, as anyone can have temporary pathological symptoms in response to a crisis.

The theories presented in this section are based on crisis theory (James & Gilliland, 2017) and contain elements of psychoanalysis, adaptational, interpersonal, chaos, and systems theory. There is also a discussion of key theories that have contributed to our understanding of the crisis. In his psychodynamic theory, Caplan's (1964) contributions to crisis theory emphasize the subjective aspects of crises. The subjective definition is the result of a perceived imbalance between the demanding occurrence and the individual's available resources. According to Caplan (1964), physical or psychological hazards activate an individual's coping or problem-solving abilities in order to restore balance. Due to the fact that humans are continually seeking balance have yet to achieve it, this imbalance emerges as disequilibrium resulting in pain.

Psychodynamic theory: According to psychodynamic theory, mourning requires the individual to let go of his or her attachment/interpersonal bond with the deceased. At its foundation, a psychoanalytic approach to mourning depends on the client's ability to comprehend their post-crisis disequilibrium through the access and processing of unconscious thoughts and past emotional experiences—a very intraindividual experience (Fine, 1980).

Adult Adaptation to Changes: In a 1981 essay, Schlossberg (1961) examined adult adaptation to change and made a connection between her proposed model and Lindemann's (1965) research of Cocoanut Grove survivors. Schlossberg rejects the term "crisis" due to its "negative connotations," preferring instead the phrase "transitions." Rogers' humanistic idea of the individual forms the groundwork for interpersonal theory. Fundamentally, individuals experiencing a crisis undergo inconsistency and a decline in positive self-esteem and self-worth.

Chaos theory has been used in a wide variety of subjects, ranging from the order of the universe to weather patterns and mathematics problems. This idea is based on evolution, which states that order arises from chaos when spontaneity, creativity, and collaboration are present (Oestreicher, 2007). In the 1960s, Bowen (1966) applied systems thinking to families and founded family systems theory, which views the family as an emotional unit. A major focus of theory is on the client's life and the crisis event or events and the return to normalcy that occurs after the event(s) that occurred.

Related stress, also referred to as mental or emotional strain was characterized by Hans Selye (1979) as a biologically grounded response pattern. Selye defined stress as a defensive mechanism that occurs in three stages: alert, resistance, and tiredness. Prolonged and severe stress has an effect on an individual's adaptability and health.

The COVID-19 spread throughout the world has been declared a global pandemic due to its rapid spread and high fatality rate. The impact of this pandemic on the current economic and political leadership is enormous (Akon & Rahman, 2020).

Realism's statist worldview has risen to prominence, and that the situation ensuing from COVID-19 only confirms Realism's assertion that states remain the primary actors in international affairs. Citizens in every country are looking to their governments to help with the issue rather than non-state entities. The 'global struggle' against COVID has been driven by states, the engines of a 'global fight.' Although the military security issue (as championed by Rationalism) has taken a back seat, environment and health security issues are almost plaguing political leaders and policymakers, the states' dominance, state borders, state rights, and border controls appear to loom large. When the logical proposed research fails, experts in international relations (IR) often resort to the constructive paradigm to explain global events differently (Ullah et al., 2020). Everything in IR, constructivists believe, is an intentional production of the countries and the individuals who make them up.

According to constructivism, the COVID epidemic originated within the Chinese mindset, manifested in a Wuhan clinical laboratory, and eventually appeared as a global pandemic. It produced anarchy when the global regulatory authorities did nothing to stop the pandemic from escalating to these deadly levels. However, the current theory does not provide any plausible explanations for how the post-COVID world order might emerge (Akon & Rahman, 2020; Pal, 2020). It is almost certain that the world will have to be dealing with the COVID-19 epidemic i.e., we will have to live with it and its long-term consequences for years to come.

Some believe that the current COVID-19 epidemic has given China fresh hope for world leadership. If China bolsters its support for developing nations while still being positive towards global governance, the global order may be reshaped, and COVID-19 may pave the way for China to rule the post-COVID-19 world order. However, China's socialist system of government may make it more difficult for the country to achieve its goals in the post-COVID-19 international society. The severity of the current outbreak may provide insight into the possibility, even though it is far too early to predict the international order following COVID-19. Post-COVID-19, the world will either witness the emergence of new world power- China, to dominate global affairs, or the balance of power will shift in favour of China. We found that globalization's de facto and de jure economic and political components had the most significant impact on policy implementation timelines. Travel restrictions are more likely to be imposed if neighbouring nations (which receive non-resident tourists) do the same. The likelihood of a government establishing a more stringent global travel policy is three times greater. Let us assume there is an alternative policy in place. These findings emphasize the connection between preventative measures and globalization measures as states respond to significant global circumstances like the current COVID-19 outbreak (Bickley et al., 2021).

When countries respond to a major worldwide epidemic, such as a public health issue, scientists point out the dynamic interplay between globalization and protectionism. Globalization's reluctance to enact policy is, we argue, owing to adherence to current trade agreements in regions with strong government efficacy. As a result, people are more likely to "learn from others" and lose faith in a government's ability to deal with an outbreak in the healthcare sector in order to find out if the globalization index may improve global infection forecasts while taking into account the critical function of government efficacy, more research is needed. By functioning as proxies for a country's likelihood and timeliness of implementing travel restriction measures, these variables could anticipate delays in initial infection and transmission across national borders.

In the long and near term, the "social economy" appears to have been vital in resolving and decreasing the COVID-19 issue's economic and social implications. With their inventive suggestions for strengthening public services and government action, social economy participants help the recovery from the crisis in the short term. The post-crisis economy can be reshaped by social economy programs that advocate for more sustainable business structures. Models of social creativity and purpose can be generated by the market economy by drawing on experience, special features, and fundamental principles (OECD, 2020a). The spread of the COVID-19 outbreak, local lockdown, the severity of the illness, inadequate healthcare governance and facilities, a lack of understanding, and the dissemination of misinformation in the media all drive public panic.

The social economy may play a prominent role in building a more effective and equitable economy and society in the post-COVID era. The social economy has shown to be a trailblazer in identifying and implementing alternative economic structures and social innovations. These inventions have been mainstreamed and embraced by the overall economy (fair trade, organic food deportment, or equitable finance). These breakthroughs aided economic and social change and will be critical in the post-COVID era.

The COVID-19 pandemic swept throughout the community, worsening the healthcare situation, creating economic hardship, and culminating in a GDP loss. The loss of their livelihoods has exacerbated people's mental and socioeconomic insecurity. In order to alleviate public concern and anxiety, the government should conduct an appropriate risk assessment, communication, and fiscal stimulus measures, as well as take suitable actions to improve mental health and well-being (Bodrud-Doza et al., 2020). According to the OECD (2020a), the focus on sustainable economic processes distinguishes the social economy: by responding to society (i.e. environmental or social) needs; by structuring economic activity around local roots and employing participatory and democratically leadership; and by collaborating closely with other sectors of the economy. There has never been a more significant need for social economy services than in current times. Economic system organizations have proven to be trustworthy partners, functioning on the front lines of the crisis to provide critical sanitary and social demands. Like other economic actors, they are feeling the effects of the lockdown, including a decline in revenue. Certain sociocultural economic legal forms (such as associations or foundations) may preclude businesses from receiving government aid during the crisis. The COVID-19 quandary needs a rebalancing of efficiency and resilience in the economy. The social economy was traditionally supposed to be utilized to "fix" societal ills (such as shelterless, labour market boycott and other forms of social exclusion experienced by vulnerable groups).

WHO (2020b) outlined a six-point framework for states considering lifting a lockdown or restriction: (1) Infection rate is controlled; (2) the health service can

The Foundation of Crisis Models

"identify, test, segregate, treat, track, and detect every infection specific instance and detect every specific instance"; (3) risk factors for vulnerable selected locations, such as healthcare facilities, are minimized; and (4) preventive measures for academic institutions are established; (5) the capability for new cases to be started importing can be regulated; and (6) the potential for new infections can be controlled.

The choice, of course, is difficult to make about lifting lockdown. Because the choice, in fact, is between life and economy. Lockdown is a way of thwarting the spread of the virus, but at the same time, it cripples the economy. However, relieving the lockdown too soon can increase the infection rate, but following the six points prescribed by the WHO does not guarantee COVID-19 infections will not resurface. Consequently, the International Labor Organization (ILO, 2020) recommends prioritizing the protection of laborers and their families from disease. Demand-side strategies to protect those who incur income losses due to infection or decreased economic activity are required to stimulate the economy. Low-wage and economically disadvantaged workers are more likely to report suspected illnesses if they have income security.

In response to the COVID-19 problem, the social-democratic critique of neoliberalism is at the heart of the competing responses. Socially progressive public healthcare, democracy and state intervention encounter anti-statists on both the left and right wing. On the link between science and governance, change theories and alternative social structures, this is a common topic of discussion. The pandemic-induced crisis is a fight between democratic, socialist and neoliberal ideas of various forms of society. The effects of healthcare, economy, politics, and violence are felt throughout society. Business leaders are also finding it difficult to respond due to the massive scale of the outbreak and its unpredictability. Indeed, the epidemic bears all of the hallmarks of a "landscape-scale" disaster: an unusual incident or series of events on numerous scales and at a quick pace, resulting in increased ambiguity, confusion, a sense of loss of control, and intense emotional distress (D'Auria & Smet, 2020).

Inequalities have implications for shaping COVID-19 transmission routes. Some particular kind of profession provides forms of interaction suitable for contracting the virus. This is critical because COVID-19 spreads by contact with contaminated things and droplets in the air. As a result, the only non-pharmaceutical treatments are now available and need considerable separation of infected and non-infected people. It is vital to achieving isolation in order to diminish and eventually eliminate the virus. Distancing is challenging since not all viral carriers exhibit symptoms, and testing for the infection is complicated. As a result, engagement with those at risk of contracting the virus and those who are already sick is critical (Obrenovic et al., 2020; Walby, 2021).

The COVID-19 pandemic created a massive system shift, connecting businesses, customers, associations, and even government in a complex web of interwoven relationships, resulting in a new ecosystem in which it became evident that no single organization could manage the ramifications the pandemic is leaving with us. In the face of the pandemic, new networked economic systems are rooted in sociotechnical systems in which environmental, community, technical, and economic values must be balanced.

COVID-19 has exacerbated some pre-pandemic issues in achieving sustainable development, the most prominent of which is the international system's frailty and inability to respond to crises. One sign of this trend is the seeming schism in the interaction between procedural actors and knowledge actors in sustainable development governance. At the regional, national and global levels, process stakeholders drive official and organizational activities and procedures (Basu et al., 2022; Bhattacharya & Khan, 2021).

COVID-19 has the potential to exacerbate poverty and inequality. While some segments of the workforce in many countries are untouched economically by the epidemic — for example, those working remotely in stable professions with full pay—those in temporary, informal, or precarious employment are frequently the hardest hurt. Many of these jobs got vanished forever, and in many cases, there is no social safety net to help newly unemployed people maintain the income close to pre-pandemic levels. With nothing to look forward to, those who have lost everything can be an easy target for political influence and radicalism (Rohner, 2020). Prior to the COVID-19 epidemic, democracy has been under significant strain, with global democracy scores showing negative trends over the last decade (Laurent-Lucchetti et al., 2020). It's possible that COVID-19 could exacerbate this trend (Rohner, 2020). Conflict theory's primary premise has frequently been confirmed by empirical evidence, showing a strong correlation between poverty and conflict and political violence (Collier et al., 2009). In canonical conflict models, poverty, a lack of human capital, and a lack of economic possibilities all serve as fertile breeding grounds for conflict (Hirshleifer, 2001). A person who is poor, desperate, and destitute is more likely to leave a job and engage in violence (Rohner, 2020).

The concentration of poverty is increasing in middle-income, fragile, and conflict-affected countries, for example, in Sub-Saharan Africa. Strict containment policies may have a detrimental effect on underprivileged regions of the world. Impoverished African households, for instance, having little financial and food resources, are rarely able to work remotely, and rely on daily labour payments. As a result, they run the risk of falling into extreme poverty if they are stranded during a lockdown and fail to return to work (Bargain, & Aminjonov, 2021).

Poverty is evolving globally. In 2020, Sub-Saharan Africa accounted for 64% of the poor, while South Asia 21%. If all goes according to plan, extreme poverty in South Asia could be eliminated by 2030. However, numerous underprivileged households have been pushed back into poverty as a result of the pandemic. Meanwhile, as a result of continued population increase and sluggish economic growth, Sub-Saharan Africa may account for 84% of the world's impoverished (Homi, 2020). Individuals have lost employment and livelihoods as a result of lockdowns and social distancing practices, leaving them unable to pay rent or feed. Schools have been closed, and some students may not return, obliterating one of the only avenues for low-income children to escape poverty. School closures have disproportionately disadvantaged women and girls (Homi, 2020).

Developing and under-developed countries find it more difficult than developed countries to implement notoriously difficult measures to deal with the COVID-19 challenge (Loayza, 2020). They may have to rely on simple relief and recovery strategies, such as making direct money transfers and assuring the continuity for public goods and services, to minimize the effects of the incident through economic policies. Governments in developing nations may need to implement public health programmes to control the disease's spread. For starters, it does not require a high level of governmental compliance responsiveness; rather, it relies on social compliance and home action. Second, it provides the supplementation of assistance from non-profit groups, the corporate sector, and international organizations. Public health initiative modelling is also becoming more realistic. Early models let governments impose indiscriminate lockdowns that differed only in length and population size. More modern models enable governments to distinguish across sectors (allowing essential activities to keep going while restricting a fraction of non-essential activities). Implement differential lockdowns or sheltering of susceptible populations (recognizing evidence that the elderly and ill are the most affected by the virus); and conduct testing, finding, and isolating infected people. These models incorporate political economy components in a number of ways.

One approach is to acknowledge the distributional implications of blanket quarantines, which benefit and hurt different segments of society in different ways. Longer, tougher lockdowns, for example, would benefit the elderly more than the youth. Another way to incorporate political and economic factors is to recognize that cooperation with mitigation and suppression measures influences the selection of acceptable human distancing. Mitigation and entrenchment measures, for example, must be milder in low allegiance circumstances. A third way highlights the feedback loops that exist between good economic strategy and motives to comply with rules. People will support temporary shutdowns if they believe the economy will recover and their jobs will be restored.

The pandemic's global scope and gradual progression clearly distinguish it from other natural calamities that have disrupted combat situations in the past. The pandemic's character also makes it impossible to see it as a window of opportunity for peace. Domestic and international peace processes suffer while the world's attention remains focused on the pandemic (Mustasilta, 2020). Again, Loayza (2020) contends that, first, in emerging than developed countries, social welfare losses owing to economic contraction are expected to be greater than all those due to fatalities. This is because of the fact that the majority of the populations in developing-country are young. Second, compliance with stringent limitations is almost certainly lower in developing countries than in developed countries. This is due to lesser perceived advantages from compliance, limited government enforcement, decreased community trust, and weaker financial relief and recovery measures. As a result, mitigation and suppression strategies in emerging countries should be less stringent and time-consuming than in developed countries. Third, because economic losses in low-income countries significantly impact their welfare, getting cost-effective pandemic-fighting steps is crucial, possibly even more so than in advanced countries. The ability to implement is a fourth complicated stage. Some "smart" mitigation strategies that could bring benefits (such as safeguarding the vulnerable and diagnosing and isolating the sick) are difficult to execute even in prosperous countries. In developing countries, their implementation is projected to be more difficult; yet, implementing "smart" measures is the only long-term option in the absence of vaccines. It will take a combination of creativity in implementing "smart" approaches, increased effort by government officials, and the community aid.

Expats and their children are disproportionately affected by the COVID-19 situation (OECD, 2020b). Due to several vulnerabilities such as greater poverty rates, congested housing conditions, and a focus on the job where physical separation is near impossible, immigrants are at a significantly higher risk of COVID19 infection than native-born people. In most OECD countries, research has indicated that infection risk is at least twice as high for foreign-born people as it is for native-born people. COVID-related death rates in immigrants may be much greater than in the native-born population.

According to studies (such as Ullah et al., 2020), discrimination increases rapidly in a weak labour market, while contact links—which migrants have less of—become increasingly vital for gaining work. Immigrants' poor labour market performance is exacerbated by the fact that they are overrepresented in the industries that have been hardest hit by the epidemic. As an example, in the hospitality business, foreign-born workers make up a quarter of all EU employees, which is more than double their share of total employment. substantial obstacles to growth are believed to have resulted from the outbreak. This year, income growth in rising sectors and developing economies is forecast to be 4.9%, but in low-income nations, the rate of increase is expected to be the same as in 2013. Three-quarters of unstable and conflict-affected low-income countries will not fully recover by 2022, according to a new report. Approximately 100 million people are predicted to return to extreme poverty by the end of 2021, according to estimates. More than half of those affected by these negative consequences are children and women, as well as those who lack the skills or organization to organize themselves. According to Arendt (2020), women and girls are routinely affected during disasters. Recognizing the gender-specific feature of pandemics is crucial for boosting COVID-19 responses at the national, regional, and global levels.

COVID-19 and its harmful repercussions can be impacted in a variety of ways by social deprivation and disaster vulnerability at the community level (Melvin et al., 2020). Lower socioeconomic status (SES), for example, is associated with reduced access to health care, which may increase the chance of adverse health outcomes. Workplace inequalities, a lack of worker safety, and overcrowding may make it challenging to adhere to social-distancing norms. The impact of such issues is amplified in rural racial and ethnic groupings. A shrinking population, economic stagnation, physician and other medical provider shortages, a disproportionate number of poor, elderly, and uninsured individuals, and high rates of chronic sickness are all variables that contribute to the problems in rural areas. Following the dread and anxiety that emerge during an epidemic, stigma and prejudice emerge quickly, exposing hatred and violence, harassment, and isolation, limiting the delivery and adoption of required healthcare services and public wellness measures to manage the pandemic.

Race, financial position, occupation, gender, immigrant status and sexual orientation could be compounded by pandemic stigma. HIV, the Ebola and Zika virus outbreaks as well as COVID-19 have all exposed the stigma associated with the underlying disease. Fear of stigmatization during a pandemic may limit the deployment of prevention measures, rapid testing, and treatment adherence. Since the discovery of COVID-19, there have been numerous forms of stigmatization and prejudice. Some countries' xenophobia has been directed at anyone suspected of carrying COVID-19 into the country. These employees are crucial because they have returned from their COVID-19 experiences refreshed and rejuvenated.

Healthcare workers and people from stigmatized and discriminated-against groups (e.g., HIV-positive people, people from sexual and gender minorities, sex workers, refugees) have all been exposed to physical and verbal abuse. Individuals living with HIV (Chattoraj et al., 2021; Ullah & Huque, 2014), particularly adolescents, women, and transgender individuals, are being forced to disclose their HIV status when attempting to receive HIV care in a number of nations during lockdowns. There has been an increase in violence among persons and women from sexual and gender minorities as a result of stay-at-home orders and physical distancing measures. Attacks on lesbian, homosexual, bisexual, and transgender adolescents have been documented under the guise of community health enforcement operations, as has a lack of social and financial security for sex workers.

According to Donnelly et al. (2021), at the height of the epidemic, 45 countries in Central Asia and Europe suspended their educational facilities, affecting 185 million students. Teachers and administrators were taken off guard by the issue's suddenness and were forced to build emergency virtual learning systems. One disadvantage of remote learning is the lack of physical contact between teacher and learner. On the other hand, several countries have taken the initiative to expand the remote learning environment by utilizing diverse technologies such as social media, email, cellphones, and the post office.

Public health and global economies face an era-defining threat from the COVID-19 pandemic, but its impact on violent conflict is less well recognized. While much is unknown, the epidemic's potential to affect vulnerable countries, foment discontent, and destabilize international crisis management mechanisms has been established (ICG, 2020). Many people expected that the scenario would lead to ceasefires in most of the world's conflicts. However, these hopes were largely dashed because of the coronavirus, conflict actors' incentive structures, possibilities, and timescales have all transformed. In some instances, violence escalated as organizations took advantage of the opportunity to ramp up their operations, primarily because state troops were preoccupied with the health issue. In other cases, non-state players seeking greater legitimacy attempted to buy local support by delivering "better pandemic governance" than their official counterparts. In certain cases, violence escalated as organizations took advantage of the opportunity to ramp up their operations, primarily because state troops were preoccupied with the health issue. In other cases, non-state players seeking greater legitimacy attempted to buy local support by delivering "better pandemic governance" than their official counterparts (Kishi, 2021).

In some countries, the epidemic's effects indirectly boosted rivalry among armed organizations, while in others, previously warring armed groups banded together to oppose the government's reaction to the outbreak. In certain cases, the coronavirus caused destruction on the political scene, escalating long-standing disputes. Nwankwo (2021) shows how a person's political and social connection can influence political activity during a pandemic. According to the study, quarantining or other connected measures, such as self-isolation, social distancing, or house confinement, are not essential because the majority of people do not believe the virus is real. People's political skepticism has a significant influence on their outlook. People who are most inclined to participate, according to the findings, do not have these attitudes and do not trust the government.

As a result, people who believe COVID-19 is real and separate themselves socially are more likely to have limited social involvement with their friends and relatives. This implies that people's attitudes can be affected by their encounters with one another, as neighbours and friends can influence one another's views on the topic, resulting in their proclivity to vote. As a result, those who believe the disease is real and adhere to COVID-19 safety requirements by quarantining will likely engage less with their neighbours and friends, potentially leading to political and social alienation impacts on their involvement disposition. However, because the majority of people feel the virus is not absolute and do not trust the government, Nigerian voter turnout is low. People who trust the government and are more likely to vote would instead not vote than contract the virus.

So according to Shammi et al. (2021), developing countries must work together to address COVID-19's impact on food security and rising poverty in light of the global economy's crisis, job losses, and a lack of RMG exports and incoming remittances. While the lockdown is lifted, both lives and livelihoods are in peril, which is the topic of a long-running debate. Along with epidemic related illness, the upcoming seasons of natural risks such as cyclones, flash floods, tidal floods, and landslides during monsoon seasons should be taken into consideration when planning for crises.

Pandemic Governance and Security Approach

Global politics draws on a variety of disciplines in the social sciences and humanities. How do we define and measure power? Is the allocation of economic and military resources sufficient to determine system polarity and predominance positions? Should we examine other, more nebulous definitions of power? Can ideas like soft, structural, agenda-setting, and institutional power assist us in better understanding international life? Are power, sovereignty, legitimacy, interdependence, justice, human rights, liberty, equality, development globalisation, inequality, sustainability, peace, conflict, violence, non-violence and international relations important in handling the pandemic?

The growing interest in the concept of global governance, as well as the reality that many theoretical frameworks have conceptualized global governance differently, make the questions of how the concept may be utilized to explain the current global order intriguing. International Relations (IR) theory has "created a formidable barrier to an IR theory" and contributed to doubts about the discipline's ability to explain changes in an increasingly complex world order, especially given that evidence appears to support conflicting theories equally and evidence varies in interpretation between theories.

To address the aforementioned concerns, this section argues that, while numerous IR theoretical paradigms emphasize distinct aspects of global governance, no single paradigm has been able to capture the intricacies of global governance. As a result, conceiving global governance requires a unique combination of realism, institutionalism, constructivism, and pluralism. While each of these theoretical frameworks is flawed in and of itself, when combined, they significantly add to our understanding of power, order, norms, and change in the global order. As a result, for global governance to become a more comprehensive and sophisticated area, IR as science must acquire the capacity to transcend restrictive theoretical restrictions.

Figure 2.1 shows the interplay between COVID-19 and the components (global governance and international development cooperation, political conflicts between states, immigration, public health, discrimination and stigma, the economy, gender vulnerability, access to education, political participation and citizen's trust) of global politics.

Political institutions influence policy initiatives and outcomes in a variety of ways. Institutions facilitate relevant players' access to decision-making processes, guide actors' preferences and opportunities, and may even influence actors' interaction (Scharpf, 1997). Varied government systems might provide different opportunities for politicians to gain credit and avoid blame for specific outcomes (Hinterleitner, 2018; Nelson, 2016). Most activities addressing the prevention and moderation of the adverse effects of pandemics, such as retrenchment policies, affect a large number of people (if not everyone) without providing immediate benefits. Prevention policies are costly (in terms of public funds).

Furthermore, as a result of the pandemic, individual liberty and rights are frequently constrained. Politicians in democratic regimes rely on public support and, as a result, avoid contentious actions (Weaver, 1986). In terms of blame avoidance, distinct expectations emerge when comparing France and Germany, which have opposing democratic orientations (Lijphart, 2012). In the French unitary majoritarian system, the president of the state (and leader of the majority party) is at the core of every decision, at least when there is no political cohabitation. As a result, the French President finds it extremely difficult to avoid taking credit for unpopular and ineffectual policies. Furthermore, public rejection and protest against unpopular policies feature French protest culture.

Digital Divide and Growing Disparity

The COVID-19 pandemic was marked by unparalleled technological development and utilization (Giansanti & Velcro, 2021). The epidemic has significantly exacerbated this situation. For the first time, millions have been forced to rely on the internet

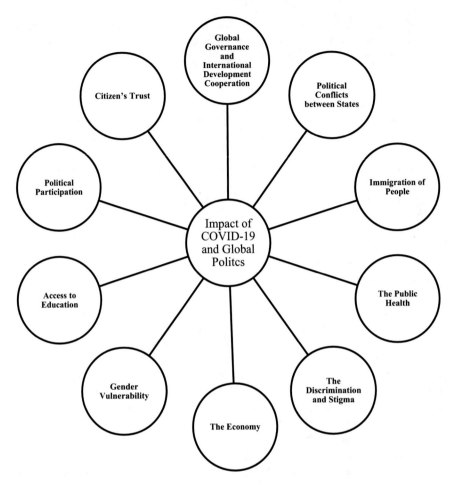

Fig. 2.1 The interplay between COVID-19 and global politics (*Sources* Developed by authors based on Arendt, 2020; Bhattacharya & Khan, 2021; Bodrud-Doza et al., 2020; Donnelly et al., 2021; Kishi, 2021; Loayza, 2020; Melvin et al., 2020; Nwankwo, 2021; Obrenovic et al., 2020; Shammi et al., 2021; UNAIDS, 2020; Walby, 2021; WHO, 2020; World Bank, 2021)

and digital devices to seek assistance, finish activities, and participate fully in society (Centre for Better Ageing, 2021).

The global crisis brought on by the coronavirus outbreak has driven us even more into a digital environment, and behavioural alterations are likely to have long-term effects when the economy recovers. However, not everyone is prepared to embrace a digital lifestyle (UNCTAD, 2020). UNCTAD investigates how certain people profit more than others from a technologically advanced world and found that the coronavirus outbreak has accelerated the usage of digital solutions, tools, and services, hastening the global shift to a digital economy. It has, however, shown the wide disparity between the connected and the unconnected, revealing how far behind many people are in terms of digital adoption (UNCTAD, 2020). Inequalities in digital readiness impede the ability of vast swaths of the world to profit from technology that allows us to stay at home and deal with the coronavirus epidemic (UNCTAD, 2021).

Let's not forget the fact that about four billion people (more than half of the global population) still have no access to the internet (UN, 2020). An example of the epidemic's effect on the digital divide was provided by Emily and her colleagues (2020) in their study that some 21% of homebound children's parents fear they won't be unable to complete their schoolwork because there is no computer at home, or because they would be forced to use public Wi-Fi because they do not have a reliable internet connection at home (22%) (Emily et al., 2020). Low-income parents have additional concerns about their children's education. When their children's schools close, many low-income parents worry that their children will be forced to complete schoolwork using only their cellphones. Forty percent of parents worry that their children will be forced to use public Wi-Fi because their home internet connection is unreliable. Roughly a third of parents worry that their children will be unable to complete schoolwork altogether (36%) (Emily et al., 2020).

By gender: According to a recent study done in Ethiopia, India (Andhra Pradesh and Telangana), Peru, and Vietnam, a widening digital divide and interrupted education worsen existing disparities (Ford, 2021). Due to the pandemic's increased reliance on information technology to combat COVID-19 and maintain economies, the pandemic will significantly increase the cost of digital exclusion for the one billion women and their families who currently do not use the internet. If males have better access to digital alternatives that preserve livelihoods and health than females, ignoring the gender digital divide exacerbates gender inequality (USAID, 2020). To combat the virus's spread, health care information (especially on COVID-19), education, and economic activities have been moved online. Internet services have increased in popularity by 40–100%, however, many people stay alienated from the online world (Aggarwal, 2020). By the age of about 15, 81% of Ethiopian rural youth had never used the internet. In India, girls from the poorest households and rural areas are disproportionately disadvantaged, with 89% of rural girls not having used the internet by the age of 15, compared to only 34% of urban boys. Even in Vietnam, where overall internet availability is high, a quarter (25%) of the poorest children had never used a computer by the time they reached the age of 15, compared to only 3% of the wealthiest children (Ford, 2021).

The digital divide is emerging as the new face of inequality, prejudice, and socioeconomic marginalization in our post-pandemic society and economy. Additionally, it is highly gendered, mirroring women's persistent exclusion from critical infrastructure. Asia is not exempt from this trend (Aggarwal, 2020). In South Asia, the gender disparity in mobile internet use was 51% in 2019. This imbalance has resulted in women and persons who identify as non-binary experiencing a lack of access to lifesaving information and services. Women received 15% less information than men in Bangladesh and Pakistan in order to escape the COVID-19 pandemic (Aggarwal, 2020).

By rich and poor: Numerous studies have found a correlation between higher internet and mobile use and increased productivity and employment (International Telecommunication Union, 2012). The digital economy anticipated being valued at approximately USD11.5 trillion in 2016 (15.5% of global GDP) (Huawei & Oxford Economics, 2017). By 2025, it is expected to account for 25% of global GDP, generating new economic opportunities. However, only half of the world's population has internet access, with connections in parts of South Asia and Sub-Saharan Africa falling to less than 30% (Huawei & Oxford Economics, 2017). Almost 2.4 billion people in the Asian Infrastructure Investment Bank (AIIB) region lack access to the internet, the majority of whom live in India, China, Indonesia, Pakistan and Bangladesh. As a result, many of these countries would struggle to harness digital technology in order to overcome economic difficulties caused by lockdowns and social estrangement and regain access to basic commodities and services. Due to the disparity in internet coverage, people across the world have experienced varying degrees of disruption in their communities as a result of the epidemic. Due to various access and adaptation restrictions, people of the majority of low-income economies are equally, unequally, or most disrupted by the COVID-19 pandemic.

By rural and urban: The expanding digital divide between the "haves" and the "have nots" has been blamed for widening income gaps within and across countries. Most emerging nations have exhibited a preference for unequal development between urban and rural areas long before the current wave of ICT developments. Urban bias is the term economists tend to use to describe this phenomenon. For a long time, those who contended that the digital divide was a "non-issue" or merely another symptom of the existing urban bias were quick to dismiss any discussion of it (Henry, 2019). More than only the availability of an accelerated catalyst is required for the expansion of the information society. To reap the benefits of information and communications technology, the general public must have both access to and expertise with these tools. COVID-19 pandemic, on the other hand, revealed the seriousness of digital vulnerability in these three dimensions: interconnection, use, and exploitation. The pandemic created an environment where internet access appears to be essential for survival, particularly in terms of health issues (De et al., 2020; Esteban-Navarro et al., 2020).

Conclusions

The most serious risks that lie ahead are overcorrection or under-correction in response to COVID-19. A complete swing back from the 1990s hyper-globalization to a strong nationalist and protectionism regime in the 2020s would be an over-correction risk. In the 1990s, proponents of globalization may have been condemned for providing an unduly rosy picture of development. They stressed the numerous and diverse benefits of globalization, depicting expanding links as both necessary and helpful. Despite the fact that shocks like the global economic crisis and COVID-19 show numerous systemic risks connected with globalization, the goal is not to believe

Conclusions

that everything domestic is good, but everything global is awful. A more measured and calibrated approach is required (Bishop & Roberts, 2020). The pandemic has the potential to radically alter global order and upend the rules-based international system established by the United States and its allies following World War II.

Rivalry among the world's most powerful nations has heated up. The global economy is in its deepest slump since the Great Depression, and social uprisings fuelled by political grievances and financial insecurity have swept the globe. The current situation needs fast and decisive action in order to emerge from the crisis and build a better future. As a result of this disaster, the powerful states and other like-minded countries can endeavour to rebuild, revitalize, and adapt a rules-based system. If they do not, others will construct a system that is harmful to the free world. The powerful countries taking up global leadership will benefit individuals all throughout the world. By addressing the vulnerabilities exposed and exploited by the virus, the United States and other like-minded countries can resurrect a rules-based system that exceeds the first in assisting individuals in achieving life, liberty, and happiness (Cimmino et al., 2020).

Suppose we assume that a worldwide reaction is to be carried out. In that instance, the fiscal space required to maintain the economy while keeping major sectors of the population at home emphasizes the need for multilateral capability extending beyond specific nation-states' individual strengths. The numerous stages of the COVID-19 pandemic, such as outbreak, lockdown, containment, and re-opening, involve coordination, and those with the least policy space require help from international organizations. Finally, an inherent clash between borderless phenomena and a political process relies on and legitimizes boundaries as defensive mechanisms (Blanco & Rosales, 2020).

COVID-19 has shown that many countries rely on international supply chains, putting them in danger in the event of a pandemic. However, there are risks associated with reshoring production. If a country is completely self-sufficient in medical supplies, a natural disaster may devastate that capacity, and imports would not be available in time to replace local production. As a result, the cost of producing drugs would rise, perhaps resulting in the loss of life at other times. Interdependence can be handled by carefully distributing exposure and combining domestic and international suppliers. These are critical concerns that must be addressed. They all demand a response that prevents relapse into pre-pandemic conditions. The major opportunity presented by COVID-19 appears to be to reconsider some of the financial approaches to better the possibilities of developing more sustainable and resilient globalization alternatives. Innovation and adaptation are crucial when dealing with global disasters that affect everyone, such as epidemics and climate change. These are the most important areas for collective action, yet they are also the most difficult to achieve.

A virus is an excellent equalizer since no country is immune to it, even if not everyone is equally exposed to or damaged by it. Because the connection is only as strong as its weakest link, the crisis would focus on efficiently assisting the most vulnerable individuals and countries. Because of our interdependence, if the vulnerable are endangered, everyone is endangered (Bishop & Roberts, 2020). This outbreak will have far-reaching consequences for the rest of the planet. Our domestic and international responses will determine whether we can learn from this catastrophe and establish a more sustainable and long-term globalization policy.

References

Aggarwal, A. (2020). *How Covid-19 fuels the digital gender divide.* Retrieved from https://itforchange.net/covid-19-fuels-digital-gender-divide-FES-in-asia. Accessed 14 July 2021.

Akon, M. S., & Rahman, M. (2020). Reshaping the global order in the post covid-19 era: A critical analysis. *Chinese Journal of International Review, 2*(1), 2050006.

Andersen, K. G., Rambaut, A., Lipkin, W. I., Holmes, E. C., & Garry, R. F. (2020). The proximal origin of SARS-CoV-2. *Nature Medicine, 26*(4), 450–452.

Arendt, F. (2020, June 9). *Addressing the vulnerability of women in the COVID-19 crisis.* UN Volunteers. Retrieved from https://www.unv.org/Success-stories/addressing-vulnerability-women-covid-19-crisis. Accessed 5 Aug 2021.

Bai, H. (2020). *Who bought all the toilet paper? Conspiracy theorists are more likely to stockpile during the COVID-19 pandemic.* Retrieved from https://psyarxiv.com/z2g34/

Ball, P., & Maxmen, A. (2020, May 27). The epic battle against coronavirus misinformation and conspiracy theories. *Nature.* Retrieved from https://www.nature.com/articles/d41586-020-014 52-z. Accessed 28 July 2021.

Bargain, O., & Aminjonov, U. (2021). Poverty and COVID-19 in Africa and Latin America. *World Development, 142,* 105422. https://doi.org/10.1016/j.worlddev.2021.105422

Barro, R. J., Ursúa, J. F., & Weng, J. (2020). *The coronavirus and the great influenza pandemic: Lessons from the "spanish flu" for the coronavirus's potential effects on mortality and economic activity* (No. w26866). National Bureau of Economic Research.

Basu, A., Ketheeswaran, N., & Cusanno, B. R. (2022). Localocentricity, mental health and medical poverty in communication about sex work, HIV and AIDS among trans women engaged in sex work. *Culture, Health & Sexuality, 24*(1), 125–137. https://doi.org/10.1080/13691058.2020.181 7562

Bertin, P., Nera, K., & Delouvee, S. (2020). *Conspiracy beliefs, rejection of vaccination, and support for hydroxychloroquine: A conceptual replication-extension in the COVID-19 pandemic context.* Retrieved from https://psyarxiv.com/rz78/

Bhattacharya, D. & Khan, S. S. (2021, June 14). *Removing the wedge between process actors and knowledge actors in development cooperation: A step toward more inclusive and networked global governance.* Center for Global Development. Retrieved from https://www.cgdev.org/blog/removing-wedge-between-process-actors-and-knowledge-act ors-development-cooperation-step-toward. Accessed 30 July 2021.

Bickley, S. J., Chan, H. F., Skali, A., Stadelmann, D., & Torgler, B. (2021). How does globalization affect COVID-19 responses? *Globalization and Health, 17*(1), 1–19.

Bieber, F. (2020). Global nationalism in times of the COVID-19 pandemic. *Nationalities Papers,* 1–13.

Bishop, J., & Roberts, A. (2020). Geopolitics: Resilient and sustainable globalisation. In *The World Economic Forum,* Geneva (pp. 20–21).

Blanco, M. L., & Rosales, A. (2020). Global governance and COVID-19: The implications of fragmentation and inequality. *E-International Relations, 6.*

Bodrud-Doza, M., Shammi, M., Bahlman, L., Islam, A. R. M., & Rahman, M. (2020). Psychosocial and socio-economic crisis in Bangladesh due to COVID-19 pandemic: A perception-based assessment. *Frontiers in Public Health, 8,* 341.

References

Bogart, L. M., & Thorburn, S. (2005). Are HIV/AIDS conspiracy beliefs a barrier to HIV prevention among African Americans? *Journal of Acquired Immune Deficiency Syndromes, 38*(2), 213–218. https://doi.org/10.1097/00126334-200502010-00014. PMID: 15671808.

Bogart, L. M., Wagner, G., Galvan, F. H., & Banks, D. (2010). Conspiracy beliefs about HIV are related to antiretroviral treatment nonadherence among African American men with HIV. *Journal of Acquired Immune Deficiency Syndromes, 53*(5), 648–655.

Bonotti, M., & Zech, S. T. (2021). *Recovering civility during COVID-19.* Springer Nature.

Bowen, M. (1966). The use of family theory in clinical practice. *Comprehensive Psychiatry, 7*(5), 345–374.

Brown, F.Z., Brechenmacher, S. & Carothers, T. (2020, April 6). *How will the coronavirus reshape democracy and governance globally?* Carnegie Endowment for International Peace. Retrieved from https://carnegieendowment.org/2020/04/06/how-will-coronavirus-reshape-democracy-and-governance-globally-pub-81470. Accessed 30 July 2021.

Caplan, C. (1964). *Principles of preventive psychiatry.* Basic Books Inc.

Centre for Better Ageing. (2021). *COVID-19 and the digital divide.* Retrieved from https://ageing-better.org.uk/sites/default/files/2021-07/COVID-19-and-the-digital-divide.pdf

Chattoraj, D., Ullah, A. K. M. A., & Hossain, M. A. (2021). The COVID-19 pandemic and the travails of Rohingya refugees in the largest Bangladeshi refugee camp. In B. Doucet, van R. Melik, & P. Filion (Eds.), *Global reflections on COVID-19 and cities: Urban inequalities in the age of pandemic.* Bristol University Policy Press.

Cimmino, J., Katz, R., Kroenig, M., Lipsky, J., & Pavel, B. (2020). *A global strategy for shaping the post-COVID-19 world.* The Atlantic Council of the United States.

Collier, P., Hoeffler, A., & Rohner, D. (2009). Beyond greed and grievance: Feasibility and civil war. *Oxford Economic Papers, 61*(1), 1–27.

Cotula, L. (2021). Towards a political economy of the COVID-19 crisis: Reflections on an agenda for research and action. *World Development, 138*, 105235.

Dacombe, R. (2021). *Conspiracy theories: Why are they thriving in the pandemic?* Retrieved from https://theconversation.com/conspiracy-theories-why-are-they-thriving-in-the-pandemic-153657. Accessed 6 Aug 2021.

D'Auria, G., & Smet, A. (2020, March 13). *Leadership in a crisis: Responding to the coronavirus outbreak and future challenges.* McKinsey & Company. Retrieved from https://www.mckinsey.com/business-functions/organization/our-insights/leadership-in-a-crisis-responding-to-the-coronavirus-outbreak-and-future-challenges. Accessed 5 Aug 2021.

De', R., Pandey, N., & Pal, A. (2020). Impact of digital surge during Covid-19 pandemic: A viewpoint on research and practice. *International Journal of Information Management, 55*, 10217.

Donnelly, R., Patrinos, H. A., & Gresham, J. (2021, April 2). *The impact of COVID-19 on education—Recommendations and opportunities for Ukraine.* The World Bank. Retrieved from https://www.worldbank.org/en/news/opinion/2021/04/02/the-impact-of-covid-19-on-education-recommendations-and-opportunities-for-ukraine. Accessed 5 Aug 2021.

Douglas, K. M. (2021). COVID-19 conspiracy theories. *Group Processes & Intergroup Relations, 24*(2), 270–275.

Douglas, K. M., Sutton, R. M., & Cichocka, A. (2017). The psychology of conspiracy theories. *Current Directions in Psychological Science, 26*(6), 538–542.

Eban, K. (2021). *The lab-leak theory: Inside the fight to uncover COVID-19's origins.* Retrieved from https://www.vanityfair.com/news/2021/06/the-lab-leak-theory-inside-the-fight-to-uncover-covid-19s-origins. Accessed 5 Aug 2020.

Emily, V., Andrew, P., Lee, R., & Monica, A. (2020). *53% of Americans say the internet has been essential during the COVID-19 outbreak.* Retrieved from https://www.pewresearch.org/internet/2020/04/30/53-of-americans-say-the-internet-has-been-essential-during-the-covid-19-outbreak/. Accessed 8 Aug 2020.

Esteban-Navarro, M. Á., García-Madurga, M. Á., Morte-Nadal, T., & Nogales-Bocio, A. I. (2020, December). the rural digital divide in the face of the COVID-19 Pandemic in Europe—Recommendations from a scoping review. In *Informatics* (Vol. 7, No. 4, p. 54). Multidisciplinary Digital Publishing Institute.

Evstatieva, M. (2020, July 10). *Anatomy of a COVID-19 conspiracy theory. NPR All Things Considered.* Retrieved from https://www.npr.org/2020/07/10/889037310/anatomy-of-a-covid-19-conspiracy-theory. Accessed 7 Jan 2021.

Fernando, R., & McKibbin, W. J. (2021). Macroeconomic policy adjustments due to COVID-19: Scenarios to 2025 with a focus on Asia. In B. John, P. J. Morgan, & T. Sonobe (Eds.), *COVID-19 Impacts and policy options: An Asian perspective* (pp. 399–472). Asian Development Bank.

Ferrer, R. A., & Klein, W. M. (2015). Risk perceptions and health behavior. *Current Opinion in Psychology, 5,* 85–89.

Fine, R. (1980). Work, depression, and creativity, psychoanalytic perspective. *Psychological Reports, 46*(3_suppl), 1195–1221. https://doi.org/10.2466/pr0.1980.46.3c.1195

Ford, K. (2021). *Addressing the gender digital divide is critical to ensure no one is left behind from COVID-19.* Young Lives. https://www.younglives.org.uk/content/addressing-gender-digital-div ide-critical-ensure-no-one-left-behind-covid-19. Accessed 12 May 2021.

Galliford, N., & Furnham, A. (2017). Individual difference factors and beliefs in medical and political conspiracy theories. *Scandinavian Journal of Psychology, 58*(5), 422–428.

Geissler, E., & Sprinkle, R. H. (2013). Disinformation squared: Was the HIV-from-Fort-Detrick myth a Stasi success? *Politics and the Life Sciences, 32*(2), 2–99.

Giansanti, D., & Velcro, G. (2021, April). The digital divide in the era of COVID-19: An investigation into an important obstacle to the access to the mHealth by the citizen. In *Healthcare* (Vol. 9, No. 4, p. 371). Multidisciplinary Digital Publishing Institute. https://doi.org/10.3390/healthcare90 40371

Gingerich, D., & Vogler, J. (2021). Pandemics and political development: The electoral legacy of the black death in Germany. *World Politics, 73*(3), 393–440. https://doi.org/10.1017/S00438871 21000034

Hardy, L. J., Mana, A., Mundell, L., Neuman, M., Benheim, S., & Otenyo, E. (2021). Who is to blame for COVID-19? Examining politicized fear and health behavior through a mixed methods study in the United States. *PloS one, 16*(9), e0256136. https://doi.org/10.1371/journal.pone.025 6136

Henry, L. (2019). *Bridging the urban-rural digital divide and mobilizing technology for poverty eradication: Challenges and gaps.* Retrieved from https://www.un.org/development/desa/dspd/ wp-content/uploads/sites/22/2019/03/Henry-Bridging-the-Digital-Divide-2019.pdf

Hinterleitner, M. (2018). Policy failures, blame games and changes to policy practice. *Journal of Public Policy, 38*(2), 221–242. https://doi.org/10.1017/s0143814x16000283

Hirshleifer, J. (2001). *The dark side of the force: Economic foundations of conflict theory.* Cambridge University Press.

Homi, K. (2020). The impact of COVID-19 on global extreme poverty. *Brookings Future Development Blog.* Retrieved from https://www.un.org/development/desa/dspd/wp-content/uploads/sites/22/2021/05/KHARAS_paper1.pdf. Accessed 26 July 2021.

Huawei & Oxford Economics. (2017). *Digital spillover: Measuring the true impact of the digital economy.* Retrieved from https://www.huawei.com/minisite/gci/en/digital-spillover/files/gci_dig ital_spillover.pdf. Accessed 14 July 2021.

Imhoff, R., & Bruder, M. (2014). Speaking (un-) truth to power: Conspiracy mentality as a generalised political attitude. *European Journal of Personality, 28,* 25–43.

Imhoff, R., & Lamberty, P. (2020). A Bioweapon or a hoax? The link between distinct conspiracy beliefs about the coronavirus disease (COVID-19) outbreak and pandemic behavior. *Social Psychological and Personality Science, 11*(8), 1110–1118. https://doi.org/10.1177/194855062 0934692

References

International Crisis Group (ICG). (2020). *The Covid-19 pandemic and deadly conflict*. Retrieved from https://www.crisisgroup.org/pandemics_public_health_deadly_conflict. Accessed 10 Feb 2021.

International Labour Organization (ILO). (2020). *COVID-19 and the world of work* (1st ed.).

International Organization for Migration (IOM). (2021). *IOM strategic response and recovery plan COVID-19*. International Organization for Migration.

International Telecommunication Union. (2012). *Impact of broadband on the economy*. Retrieved from https://www.itu.int/ITU-D/treg/broadband/ITU-BB-Reports_Impact-of-Broadb and-on-the-Economy.pdf. Accessed 5 July 2021.

James, R. K., & Gilliland, B. E. (2017). *Crisis intervention strategies* (8th ed.). Cengage Learning.

Kishi, R. (2021). *A year of COVID-19: The pandemic's impact on global conflict and demonstration trends*. Retrieved from https://reliefweb.int/sites/reliefweb.int/files/resources/ACLED_A-Year-of-COVID19_April2021-compressed.pdf. Accessed 30 July 2021.

Klofstad, C. A., Uscinski, J. E., Connolly, J. M., & West, J. P. (2019). What drives people to believe in Zika conspiracy theories? *Palgrave Communications, 5*, 1–8.

Lamberty, P., & Imhoff, R. (2018). Powerful pharma and its marginalized alternatives? Effects of individual differences in conspiracy mentality on attitudes toward medical approaches. *Social Psychology, 49*(5), 255–270. https://doi.org/10.1027/1864-9335/a000347

Laurent-Lucchetti, J., Rohner, D., & Thoenig, M. (2020). *Ethnic conflicts and the informational dividend of democracy*. Retrieved from https://www.tax.mpg.de/fileadmin/TAX/docs/all/event/LRT_20Oct2020.pdf

Leman, P. J., & Cinnirella, M. (2007). A major event has a major cause: Evidence for the role of heuristics in reasoning about conspiracy theories. *Social Psychological Review, 9*, 18–28.

Lewandowsky, S., & Cook, J. (2020). *The conspiracy theory handbook*. Retrieved from https://www.climatechangecommunication.org/wp-content/uploads/2020/03/ConspiracyTheoryHandb ook.pdf. Accessed 2 July 2021.

Lewis, H. (2020. March 19). The coronavirus is a disaster for feminism. *The Atlantic*. Retrieved from https://www.theatlantic.com/international/archive/2020/03/feminism-womens-rights-coronavirus-covid19/608302/. Accessed 30 July 2021.

Lijphart, A. (2012). *Patterns of democracy: government forms and performance in thirty-six countries* (2nd ed.). Yale University Press.

Lindemann, E. (1953). Mental health fundamental to a dynamic epidemiology of health. The epidemiology of health. In I. Galdston (Ed.), *The epidemiology of health*. Health Education Council.

Loayza, N. (2020). *Costs and trade-offs in the fight against the COVID-19 pandemic: A developing country perspective*. World Bank Research and Policy Briefs (148535). Retrieved from https://www.piatafinanciara.ro/wp-content/uploads/2020/06/World-Bank-Document.pdf. Accessed 30 Sept 2021.

Lor, P., Wiles, B., & Britz, J. (2021). Re-thinking information ethics: Truth, conspiracy theories, and librarians in the COVID-19 era. *Libri, 71*(1), 1–14.

Mana, A., Bauer, G. F., Magistretti, C. M., Sardu, C., Juvinyà-Canal, D., Hardy, L. J., ... Sagy, S. (2021). Order out of chaos: Sense of coherence and the mediating role of coping resources in explaining mental health during COVID-19 in 7 countries. *SSM-Mental Health, 1*, 100001.

McLuhan, M., & Moos, M. (2014). *Media research: Technology, art and communication*. Routledge.

Melvin, S. C., Wiggins, C., Burse, N., Thompson, E., & Monger, M. (2020). Peer reviewed: The role of public health in COVID-19 emergency response efforts from a rural health perspective. *Preventing Chronic Disease, 17*. https://doi.org/10.5888/pcd17.200256

Mustasilta, K. (2020, October 23). *The effects of the COVID-19 pandemic on peace and conflict*. Retrieved from https://reliefweb.int/report/world/effects-covid-19-pandemic-peace-and-conflict. Accessed 30 July 2021.

Nelson, M. (2016). Credit-claiming or blame avoidance? Comparing the relationship between welfare state beliefs and the framing of social policy retrenchment in France and Germany. *Journal of Comparative Policy Analysis: Research and Practice, 18*(2), 138–156.

Nwankwo, C. F. (2021). COVID-19 pandemic and political participation in Lagos Nigeria. *SN Social Sciences, 1*(6), 1–23.

Obrenovic, B., Du, J., Godinic, D., Tsoy, D., Khan, M. A. S., & Jakhongirov, I. (2020). Sustaining enterprise operations and productivity during the COVID-19 pandemic: "Enterprise Effectiveness and Sustainability Model." *Sustainability, 12*(15), 5981.

OECD. (2020b). Unemployment rates, OECD—Updated: November 2020. Retrieved from http://www.oecd.org/sdd/labour-stats/unemployment-rates-oecd-update-november-2020.htm. Accessed 12 Oct 2021.

Oestreicher, C. (2007). A history of chaos theory. *Dialogues in Clinical Neuroscience, 9*(3), 279–289.

Oliver, J. E., & Wood, T. (2014). Medical conspiracy theories and health behaviors in the United States. *JAMA Internal Medicine, 174*(5), 817–818.

Organisation for Economic Co-operation and Development (OECD). (2020a). *Social economy and the COVID-19 crisis: Current and future roles.* OECD Publishing.

Organisation for Economic Co-operation and Development (OECD). (2020b). *What is the impact of the COVID-19 pandemic on immigrants and their children?* Retrieved from https://www.oecd.org/coronavirus/policy-responses/what-is-the-impact-of-the-covid-19-pandemic-on-immigrants-and-their-children-e7cbb7de/. Accessed 15 Feb 2020.

Pal, P. (2020, June 20). Managing a post-COVID global order: Looking through the lens of international relations. Extraordinary and plenipotentiary. *Diplomatist.* Retrieved from https://diplomatist.com/2020/06/20/managing-a-post-covid-global-order-looking-through-the-lens-of-international-relations/. Accessed 4 Aug 2021.

Rohner, D. (2020). Covid-19 and conflict: Major risks and policy responses. *Peace Economics, Peace Science and Public Policy, 26*(3), 20200043.

Sawada, Y., & Sumulong, L. R. (2021). Macroeconomic impacts of the COVID-19 pandemic in developing Asia. In J. Beirne, P. J. Morgan, & T. Sonobe T. (Eds). *COVID-19 impacts and policy options: An Asian perspective* (pp. 11–47). Asian Development Bank.

Scharpf, F. W. (1997). *Games real actors play: Actor-centered institutionalism in policy research.* Westview Press.

Schlossberg, N. K. (1961). *Model of counseling adults in transition.* https://www.uwyo.edu/ade d5050/5050unit4/schlossberg.asp

Selye, H. (1979). *Stress of my life: A scientist's memoirs.* Van Nostrand Reinhold Company.

Shammi, M., Bodrud-Doza, M., Islam, A. R. M. T., & Rahman, M. M. (2021). Strategic assessment of COVID-19 pandemic in Bangladesh: Comparative lockdown scenario analysis, public perception, and management for sustainability. *Environment, Development and Sustainability, 23*(4), 6148–6191.

Shinozaki, S., & Rao, L. N. (2021). Impacts of COVID-19 on micro, small, and medium-sized enterprises under lockdown: Evidence from a rapid survey in the Philippines. In J. Beirne, P. J. Morgan, & T. Sonobe (Eds.), *COVID-19 impacts and policy options: An Asian perspective* (pp. 140–187). Asian Development Bank.

Slessor, C. (2020, May 3). *Why do coronavirus sceptics and deniers continue to downplay the disease?* abcNews. Retrieved from https://www.abc.net.au/news/2020-05-03/coronavirus-sceptics-continue-to-downplay-covid19/12201344. Accessed 10 Dec 2021.

Stanley, M., Barr, N., Peters, K., & Seli, P. (2020, March 30). Analytic-thinking predicts hoax beliefs and helping behaviors in response to the COVID-19 pandemic. https://doi.org/10.31234/osf.io/m3vth. Accessed 18 Aug 2021.

The Medical Futurist. (2020, May 19). *Debunking COVID-19 conspiracy theories.* Retrieved from https://medicalfuturist.com/debunking-covid-19-theories/. Accessed 18 Sept 2021.

Ullah, A. A., Hasan, N. H., Mohamad, S. M., & Chattoraj, D. (2020). Migration and security: Implications for minority migrant groups. *India Quarterly, 76*(1), 136–153.

Ullah, A. A., Hossain, M. A., & Chattoraj, D. (2020). Covid-19 and Rohingya refugee camps in Bangladesh. *Intellectual Discourse, 28*(2), 793–806.

References

Ullah, A. A., & Huque, A. S. (2014). *Asian immigrants in North America with HIV/AIDS: Stigma, vulnerabilities and human rights.* Springer.

Ullah, A. A., Lee, S. C. W., Hassan, N. H., & Nawaz, F. (2020). Xenophobia in the GCC countries: Migrants' desire and distress. *Global Affairs, 6*(2), 203–223.

Ullah, A. K. M., Hossain, M. A., Azizuddin, M., & Nawaz, F. (2020). Social research methods: Migration in perspective. *Migration Letters, 17*(2), 357–368.

Ullah, A. A., Hasan, N. H., Mohamad, S. M., & Chattoraj, D. (2021). Privileged migrants and their sense of belonging: Insider or outsider? *Asian Journal of Social Science, 49*(3), 161–169.

Ullah, A. A., Hossain, M. A., & Huque, A. S. (2021). Non-conventional migration: An evolving pattern in South Asia. *Journal of African and Asian Studies, 56*(3), 00219096211008468.

Ullah, A. A., Kumpoh, A. A. Z. A., & Haji-Othman, N. A. (2021). Covid-19 vaccine and international relations: New frontiers of vaccine diplomacy. *Southeast Asia: A Multidisciplinary Journal, 21*(1), 1–14.

Ullah, A. A., Nawaz, F., & Chattoraj, D. (2021). *Locked up under lockdown: The COVID-19 pandemic and the migrant population. Social Sciences & Humanities Open, 3*(1), 1–5. https://doi.org/10.1016/j.ssaho.2021.100126

UN. (2020, June 28). *Against the odds: stories from women in Thailand during COVID-19.* Retrieved from https://thailand.un.org/en/51835-against-odds-stories-women-thailand-during-covid-19. Accessed 30 July 2021.

UNAIDS. (2020). *Addressing stigma and discrimination in the COVID-19 response.* Retrieved from https://www.unaids.org/sites/default/files/media_asset/covid19-stigma-brief_en.pdf. Accessed 5 Aug 2021.

UNCTAD. (2020). *Coronavirus reveals need to bridge the digital divide.* Retrieved from https://unctad.org/news/coronavirus-reveals-need-bridge-digital-divide. Accessed 6 Aug 2021.

UNCTAD. (2021, June 30). *Global economy could lose over $4 trillion due to COVID-19 impact on tourism.* Retrieved from https://unctad.org/news/global-economy-could-lose-over-4-trillion-due-covid-19-impact-tourism. Accessed 8 Aug 2021.

USAID. (2020). *USAID digital strategy.* Retrieved from https://www.usaid.gov/sites/default/files/documents/15396/COVID-19_and_Gender_Digital_Divide.pdf. Accessed 18 Aug 2021.

Van Bavel, J. J., Boggio, P., Capraro, V., Cichocka, A., Cikara, M., Crockett, M., ... Ellemers, N. (2020). *Using social and behavioural science to support COVID-19 pandemic response.* Retrieved from https://psyarxiv.com/y38m9/. Accessed 22 Aug 2021.

Van Prooijen, J. W., & Douglas, K. M. (2017). Conspiracy theories as part of history: The role of societal crisis situations. *Memory Studies, 10*(3), 323–333.

Walby, S. (2021). The COVID pandemic and social theory: Social democracy and public health in the crisis. *European Journal of Social Theory, 24*(1), 22–43.

Washington Post. (2021, May 17). *Two possible theories of the pandemic's origins remain viable. The world needs to know.* Retrieved from https://www.washingtonpost.com/opinions/global-opinions/two-possible-theories-of-the-pandemics-origins-remain-viable-the-world-needs-to-know/2021/05/17/b87f0b0e-b737-11eb-96b9-e949d5397de9_story.html. Accessed 31 Oct 2021.

Weaver, R. K. (1986). The politics of blame avoidance. *Journal of Public Policy, 6*(4), 371–398.

World Bank. (2020). *Monitoring COVID-19 impacts on households in Mongolia.* Retrieved from https://www.worldbank.org/en/country/mongolia/brief/monitoring-covid-19-impacts-on-households-in-mongolia. Accessed 1 Aug 2021.

World Bank (2021, June 8). *The global economy: on track for strong but uneven growth as COVID-19 still weighs.* The World Bank. Retrieved from https://www.worldbank.org/en/news/feature/2021/06/08/the-global-economy-on-track-for-strong-but-uneven-growth-as-covid-19-still-weighs. Accessed 5 Aug 2021.

World Health Organization (WHO). (2020a). *Impact of COVID-19 on people's livelihoods, their health and our food systems.* Retrieved from https://www.who.int/news/item/13-10-2020-impact-of-covid-19-on-people%27s-livelihoods-their-health-and-our-food-systems. Accessed 1 Aug 2021.

World Health Organization (WHO). (2020b, May 4). *WHO Bangladesh COVID-19 situation report no 10*. Retrieved from https://www.who.int/docs/default-source/searo/bangladesh/covid-19-who-bangladesh-situation-reports/who-ban-covid-19-sitrep-10.pdf?sfvrsn=c0aac0b8_4. Accessed 5 Aug 2021.

Wu, J., Cai, W., Watkins, D., & Glanz, J. (2020). How the virus got out The New York Times. *The New York Times*, 22. Retrieved from https://www.nytimes.com/interactive/2020/03/22/world/coronavirus-spread.html. Accessed 1 Aug 2021.

Zhang, L., Shen, F. M., Chen, F., & Lin, Z. (2020). Origin and evolution of the 2019 novel coronavirus. *Clinical Infectious Diseases, 71*(15), 882–883.

Chapter 3
Politicization of Pandemic and the Ramifications

Introduction

In the previous chapter, we drew on applicable concepts to explain pandemics and global politics. In this particular book, in the broadest sense, concepts and theories are one or more assumptions involving virus spread, blame games, and politics. This chapter would not have been grounded if it had not been for the prior one. Chapter 2 is crucial for readers to grasp and connect the context, previous crises with the current one the world is experiencing. This chapter examines how and why a global crisis gets politicized, as well as the implications of doing so. The perceptions of infection risk influence individuals' compliance with regulations. Several researchers have identified a link between individual-level political tendency and perceptions of COVID-19-related health risk.

Of course, there is always a political component in public health decisions. However, serious challenges occur when decisions are not built on common facts or when the science employed to analyse the situation is politicized. Such politicization of research, for example, around vaccines, can lead to policies that directly boost infection rates and damages, with perhaps fatal repercussions. History does not repeat itself, but it teaches us lessons and encourages us to respond and behave differently to address crises. Unfortunately, we do not seem to have learnt from the earlier crises; instead, we have ruthlessly politicized the current COVID-19 pandemic for political and ideological goals. This chapter discusses COVID-19's several political repercussions, including how it intensified existing political tensions within and between nations, exacerbated pre-existing international challenges connected to human mobility, and affected confidence and political activity levels.

The global pandemic has triggered a cascade of domestic and global political issues. This seems to have plagued international politics. The gap between public and private products was growing wider, and multilateralism was under attack. The COVID-19 outbreak, on the other hand, has expedited these shifts while simultaneously presenting novel opportunities to reconstruct the international pattern. COVID-19 has suddenly appeared as an external shock to the global system, reshaping global

© The Author(s), under exclusive license to Springer Nature Singapore Pte Ltd. 2022
AKM. A. Ullah and J. Ferdous, *The Post-Pandemic World and Global Politics*,
https://doi.org/10.1007/978-981-19-1910-7_3

politics and igniting new wars between adversaries and allies. It has the potential to have long-term and far-reaching geopolitical ramifications (Heisbourg, 2020). The outbreak put an end to the previously established patterns of social contact that had sustained economic and social activities. The majority of people have had their daily routines disrupted as a result of compulsory social isolation, with additional disruptions to school, work, social, and family connections possible. Organizations concerned with education, social services, health, and religion have suffered as a result. Government, criminology, and the law, as well as several other industries that rely on social contact, have been compelled to rapidly alter their mode of operations, transferring specific processes online, delaying or postponing others, and even shutting down others entirely (Felbab-Brown, 2020).

In many situations, governments have already been left urging for sufficient supplies and resources to effectively combat the Virus, putting the country's interests and the well-being of its citizens first. Most governments throughout the world have been seeking to get appropriate and necessary supplies and resources to combat the Virus in a range of conditions while balancing their national interests and citizens' well-being. When mass production began, a type of "vaccine nationalism" emerged, erecting barriers to collaboration and favouring domestic distribution (Bonotti & Zech, 2021).

In many countries, the power structure between military and civil authorities has evolved as a result of crisis responses. The army has been instructed to enforce lockdowns and help in epidemic response in a range of countries, including Iran, Peru, Israel, and South Africa. While this is almost certainly required in a crisis, it may pave the way for future military interference in domestic economic and political affairs. Crisis reactions in other regions have the potential to strengthen civilian dominance over military actors; this has already occurred. Pakistan, for example, is embroiled in a power struggle between military and civilian leaders over how to respond to the outbreak, pushing security personnel to work directly with provincial governments rather than the civilian prime minister. In order to assert control over the response, military authorities appear to have amassed enormous decision-making authority in Iran. Delegating greater enforcement functions to the military may be problematic in countries where armed forces have a history of violating human rights (Madiwale & Virk, 2011).

South Africa was initially found responsible for these problems, with army and police officials accused of deploying excessive force during the initial lockdown. Kenyan human rights organizations accused security officials of Kenya of exceeding their authority (Brown et al., 2020). It will be crucial to see if civil authorities regain control of policing and other capabilities or if the epidemic permanently increases the role of military actors in financial administration, government decision-making, and internal security. However, in countries where military troops already wield significant political power, an ineffective response could imperil their role as peacekeepers.

Overall, the outlook is bleak. However, there may be some silver linings to the pandemic's impact. Of course, civil society organizations operating on the front lines of the pandemic may contribute to the democratic vitality of the community. Effective

Introduction

state interventions may help reestablish trust in governmental or technocratic capacities in particular places. Disruptions in the voting process may spark much-needed innovation in vote management. Supporters of democracies may pay close attention to the vast array of negative and positive results in order to identify entry points and cures that can prevent long-term harm and nurture potential benefits (Brown et al., 2020).

What the History Has to Tell Us

Many people are drawing comparisons between the current COVID-19 outbreak and the influenza pandemic that swept the world less than a century ago. If this pandemic is as bad as the 1918 influenza pandemic, it will have long-term ramifications, not the least of which is the way governments deliver healthcare (Spinney, 2020). The 1918 flu pandemic claimed the lives of at least 50 million individuals or 2.5% of the world's population. There were three waves of it spreading over the world at once. After a very moderate wave in the first months of 1918, a much larger one exploded in late August. A third and final wave followed it in 1919 that was milder than the previous two waves, which passed before the end of the year. Over a 13-week span in the middle of September and December of 1918, the majority of people died. It was the worst tidal wave since the Black Death of the fourteenth century and perhaps in human history as a whole (Spinney, 2020).

Despite the fact that influenza and COVID-19 are two distinct diseases that share many similarities. Air, hands, and surfaces all have a role in the transmission of each of these diseases. Both are highly contagious viral diseases. In comparison to seasonal flu, COVID-19 kills a far larger percentage of infected individuals. However, it is unclear how it compares to pandemic influenza, which caused the 1918 calamity. When it comes to the spread of disease, both are known as "crowd diseases," which means that they thrive in situations where there are a lot of people around. Historians agree that the 1918 pandemic expedited the end of the war since both sides lost a high number of troops to the disease in the last months of the conflict.

Any kind of illness worsens human inequities. Those who live in overcrowded and impoverished settings are more vulnerable than the general population. The immune system can be weakened by malnutrition, overwork, and other underlying conditions. If they don't have access to high-quality healthcare, they are much more vulnerable. These disadvantages frequently coincide, suggesting that the poor, working-class, and those in less developed countries face the brunt of an epidemic. With this in mind, it is believed that almost a quarter of a million Indians perished from the 1918 flu, making it the deadliest pandemic in history (Spinney, 2020). For example, a huge public health campaign was launched in India in 1896, which included cleaning, fumigating, and even torching indigenous Indian dwellings. At first, they doubted that rat fleas were the source of the sickness. A better strategy would have been to examine imported commodities rather than people and to de-ratify buildings rather than clean them if they had done so (Spinney, 2020).

There was a different explanation for these anomalies in 1918. Eugenics was a commonly held notion at the time, and rich elites saw labourers and the poor as lower forms of human beings who lacked the will to improve their standard of living. As a result, if they became sick and died from diseases like typhus or cholera because of their living conditions, the causes were internal rather than external. During an epidemic, the term "public health" is frequently used to describe a coordinated attempt to shield the upper classes from the contaminating effects of the afflicted lower classes.

Blaming individuals or separating them was no longer acceptable after the 1918 disaster. Socialized medicine was a popular idea in the 1920s when several countries adopted universal healthcare that was provided at no cost to the patient. A centralized public healthcare system backed by state-run insurance was initially established in Russia, but Germany, France, and the United Kingdom swiftly followed suit. In the 1930s, the United States adopted employer-based insurance schemes, which began to thrive, but all of these countries took steps to centralize and expand access to healthcare following the flu epidemic (Spinney, 2020).

In the course of human history, there have been a number of devastating epidemics and pandemics, but which ones were the most devastating? Many pandemics have wiped out entire civilizations and brought once-mighty nations to their knees, claiming the lives of many millions of people (Jarus, 2021).

Prehistory of an epidemic: Some 5000 years ago, a disease wiped out a Neolithic hamlet in China. There were many bodies heaped up in a house that was eventually burned down. No age category was spared: skeletons of children, young adults, and middle-aged people were found. The prehistoric site, today known as "Hamin Mangha," is one of the best-preserved in China's north-eastern region, and as a result of the rapid spread of the pandemic, the land was never occupied again (Jarus, 2021).

Plague of Athens: After a five-year war between Athens and Sparta, an epidemic decimated Athens' population in 430 B.C. At least a hundred thousand people may have died. People in good health were suddenly troubled by severe heats in the head, redness and inflammation in the eyes, internal organs such as the neck or tongue glowing scarlet and producing an abnormal and fetid breath (Matta, 2020).

At this time in history, the Antonian Plague ravaged the Roman Empire: Roman legions brought back with them more than only the trophies of victory when they returned from campaigns. At least 5 million people perished from the Antonine Plague, which may have been smallpox (Matta, 2020).

The reign of Cyprian the Great: An estimated 5,000 people died per day in Rome alone during the Plague of Cyprian, which is called after St. Cyprian, a bishop of Carthage (a city in Tunisia). Researchers in Luxor, Egypt, uncovered a mass grave in 2014 that looks to be a burial ground for plague victims. Lime was smeared on their bodies in a thick layer (historically used as a disinfectant). Archaeologists uncovered three lime kilns and the charred remains of plague victims in a massive bonfire (Jarus, 2021).

Justinian's Plague: As a result of the bubonic plague, the Byzantine Empire came to an end. After that, the pandemic recurred on a regular basis. According to some estimations, as many as 10% of the world's population was wiped out (Huremović,

2019). Justinian, the Byzantine Emperor, is remembered in the pandemic's name (reigned A.D. 527–565). Alexander led the Byzantine Empire from the Middle East to Europe's farthest west (Jarus, 2021).

The black death: The Black Death spread from Asia to Europe, wreaking havoc in its wake. More than half of Europe's population was wiped out by the pandemic. Fleas on infected rats disseminate a form of Yersinia pestis that is probably no longer prevalent (Huremović, 2019; Jarus, 2021).

Cocoliztli Epidemic: More than 15 million individuals in Mexico and Central America died as a result of a viral haemorrhagic fever known as Cocoliztli. Drought-ravaged populations were devastated by the spread of a contagious disease. The Aztec term for "pest" is "Cocoliztli." Enteric fever, which includes typhoid, can be caused by S. paratyphi C, a Salmonella strain. A recent analysis confirmed this to be the case. Today, enteric fever, which can produce high fever, dehydration, and digestive issues, remains a significant public health issue (Huremović, 2019).

The American Plague: European explorers brought these diseases to the Americas, and the disease is known as the American Plagues. Inca and Aztec civilizations were decimated by smallpox and other infectious diseases. Many people believe that the indigenous peoples of the Western Hemisphere were completely wiped out. The Spanish conquest of Tenochtitlan, the Aztec capital, in 1519 was made possible by the spread of infectious diseases. Francisco Pizarro led a new Spanish expedition in 1532 that defeated the Incas. The Spanish took both empires' territories. As a result of sickness, the Aztec and Incan armies were utterly defeated on both occasions (Jarus, 2021).

London's Great Plague: King Charles II commanded a vast flight from London during the last major epidemic of the Black Death in Great Britain. The epidemic began in April 1665 and spread quickly throughout the sweltering summer months. Fleas transmitted by rats infected with the plague were a major mechanism of spread (Jarus, 2021).

Marseille's Great Plague: When a ship named "Grand-Saint-Antoine" docked in Marseille, France, carrying goods from the eastern Mediterranean, the Great Plague of Marseille was said to have begun. It is highly likely that the plague entered the city despite quarantine because of fleas on diseased animals (McDowell, 2006; Slauter, 2011).

The Russian Plague: As many as 52,000–100,000 people were killed in Moscow alone during the Russian plague pandemic, which is frequently referred to as the Plague of 1771 (Heilbronner, 1962). People's anxiety was shown in acts of violence in the plague-ravaged city of Moscow. Archbishop Ambrosius was assassinated for urging people not to attend church during the city's riots, culminating in his death (Siena, 2019).

Yellow fever in Philadelphia: Officials in Philadelphia, the capital of the United States at the time, thought that slaves were immune to yellow fever, and an anti-slavery movement advocated for the use of African-Americans to offer medical care (Rawcliffe, 2013). It was a hot and humid summer in Philadelphia that year, and mosquitoes, which carry and transmit the disease, increased in numbers.

Flu pandemic: New transportation links created by the industrial revolution have made it easier for influenza viruses to cause havoc over the world. There were one million deaths worldwide in just a few months because of the sickness. In less than five weeks, the epidemic reached its peak of death rate (Jarus, 2021).

The American Polio Epidemic: There were 27,000 cases of polio in the United States after an outbreak started in New York City. The sickness is more common among children, and some who survive it are left permanently unable to work (Porte, 1985).

Spanish Flu: More than 500 million people fell victim of the Spanish flu-one of the deadliest pandemics in human history, and with indigenous populations on the verge of extinction, the death toll is believed to be between 17 and 50 million, and maybe as high as 100 million. Soldiers' overcrowding and a subpar military diet, both of which were experienced by many civilians during World War I, aided the spread and severity of the flu. There's no evidence that the Spanish flu originated in Spain, despite its name. During World War II, Spain was a neutral country, allowing its journalists to freely disseminate early reports of the disease. Because of this, the Virus was dubbed "Spanish Flu" by many who thought it was confined to Spain (Pickstone, 1992).

Asian Flu: Another global influenza outbreak was the Asian flu pandemic. About one million people died as a result of the sickness, which was first discovered in China. Many avian influenza viruses were combined to create the pandemic virus (McDowell, 2006).

HIV/AIDS: Since its discovery in 1981, Pandemic and Epidemic Aids has claimed the lives of an estimated 35 million people. Human immunodeficiency virus (HIV), which causes AIDS, is most likely derived from a chimpanzee that spread to humans in West Africa in the early 1920s. The Virus had spread over the world by the end of the twentieth century, and AIDS had become a worldwide epidemic. More than two-thirds of the estimated 40 million persons infected with HIV reside in sub-Saharan Africa (Kreager, 1988).

H1N1 Swine Flu Pandemic: H1N1, a novel strain of swine flu that first surfaced in Mexico in the spring of 2009, soon spread throughout Europe, the United States, and Asia. Between 151,700 and 575,400 individuals died as a result of the Virus, which infected up to 1.4 billion people worldwide in a single year (Jarus, 2021).

West African Ebola Epidemic: There were 28,600 confirmed cases of Ebola in West Africa between 2014 and 2016, which resulted in 11,325 deaths. The pandemic has spread rapidly from Guinea to Liberia and Sierra Leone since December 2013. The majority of cases and deaths occurred in these three nations. According to the Centres for Disease Control and Prevention, there were fewer cases of Ebola in Africa and the US than previously reported (Jarus, 2021).

The Zika Virus Epidemic: The Zika outbreak in South and Central America will have long-term consequences. There is still a race against time as scientists work to contain the epidemic. While Aedes mosquitoes are the primary vectors of the Zika virus, it can also be transferred sexually in humans (Jarus, 2021). As the COVID-19 outbreak began, both political leaders and the general public were looking for a source of blame and a way to avoid the epidemic (Ullah, Haji-Othman, & Daud, 2021). A wide range of oppressed groups, including Asian-Americans and persons of Asian heritage, were the targets of hate crimes committed all around the world. Muslims in India, Africans in China, and Ivorians in Tunisia are among the communities who have experienced discrimination and fear of stigma as a result of the epidemic.

The pandemic has come as a source of double discrimination for some particular group of people. For example, religious, ethnic, and racial minorities and immigrants were frequently accused of being terrorists (Cohn, 2018). Discrimination and violence against people based on their race, ethnicity, or nationality were among the methods used to attack these persons (Weis, 1995), and now that the pandemic broke out, these population groups are blamed as virus carriers. "Othering" is a term used by social scientists to describe the practices of discrimination on the impoverished. There are several ways to use the method of othering, which is the practice of treating another group of people as if they are defective. A lot of attention has been devoted to anti-Chinese and anti-Asian speech, prejudice, and violence in the United States since US President Donald Trump and his administration constantly accused China—for example, coronavirus as the "China virus" or COVID-19 as the "Kung Flu" (Nakamura, 2020).

Discrimination and violence against Chinese, Chinese in the diaspora, and people of Asian descent have occurred in a number of countries. Racism against Asians has occurred on public transportation, in stores, at schools, and even when walking down the street in France (Tamara, 2020). According to the history of pandemics, we are now in a particularly risky period of time. We tend to underestimate historical hazards and calamities because we know that humanity has been able to overcome them. Despite this, previous crises appeared to be as serious and disruptive as the current ones at the time of their occurrence (Delanty, 2021). The human toll and devastation caused by epidemics of numerous diseases have been extensively chronicled for a long time.

Many people have been killed and millions have been forced to flee their homes because of this disease; it has triggered state of emergency declarations, severely restricted travel, and forced the cancellation or postponement of many elections; and it has subjected citizens to extensive and intrusive administrative control. Controversial theories have been revived, along with some political authorities' ludicrous denials of medical reality about COVID-19. The pandemic outbreak has exacerbated long-standing differences between countries, particularly those over trade and other issues between China and the United States (Roberts, 2020). An anthropologist from Canada, Wade Davis, attempted to encapsulate the political lessons of the pandemic. Assuming that vaccines would not be available for some time, he then moved on to the opinion that Canada handled the pandemic better than the United States. This belief has already been relegated to the history books (Gopnik, 2021).

It is imperative to research global governance in the health system in light of the virus's rapid growth, exacerbated by globalization. How domestic diffusion processes influence global health standards in the face of potential dangers is an issue that merits answers in light of this epidemic. We need to widen the global–local nexus in cases involving health security concerns by looking at the local's position at the global–local interface in the COVID-19 scenario (Biswas, 2021). With the

COVID-19 health risk, we emphasize the importance of national-level dissemination techniques in affecting the global health security system. That's because countries had their own self-regulatory patterns of behaviour when it came to dealing with the COVID-19 problem at the national level, notwithstanding global regulation in accordance with the WHO norms. Reiterating that national governments play an essential role in the management of epidemics and developing a health security paradigm, the COVID-19 scenario underscored the importance of resources and access to health care. The COVID-19 pandemic highlights the importance of national decision-making in establishing vital health care standards (Biswas, 2021). When faced with a massive calamity, international institutions were shown to be "fragile," leading to a shift toward economic nationalism and the comeback of state authority (Levy, 2020). As a result, there has been a rise in authoritarian populism, accompanied by intrusive government measures and a trend toward volunteer governance, spearheaded by private actors (Levy, 2020).

Reshaping Compliance

The politicization and political exploitation of pandemics is nothing new. The 1918 H1N1 flu, HIV/AIDS, and Ebola were not exempt from this rule (Adida, 2017; Cotter, 2020). People's views are shaped by the media, which are key conduits for information between decision-makers and the general population. The media's power to shape our thoughts is a testament to its impact. As an engine, our thoughts propel and guide our actions and behaviour (Abbas, 2020). According to Scott (2014), the political repercussions of disease and responses to infection are intrinsically politicized. People's compliance or noncompliance with social distancing restrictions during lockdown days is strongly affected by the politicization of COVID-19 (Russel et al., 2021).

Pandemic politicization and the dissemination of fear and hate speech result in negative and harmful discrimination and stigmatization of "others" (Cotter, 2020). Public attitudes on disease management have been affected and continue to be shaped by the politicization of diseases. Russel and colleagues (2021) found in their research that respondents with right-leaning views were shown to favour less COVID-related restrictions (Russel et al., 2021).

Toxic, often radical, political ideologies are rampant in many of the falsehoods being propagated about "public health," as well. There are many reasons for this polarization, but it also has a worldwide impact because the US's global dominance is dwindling. Still, its media, giant technological corporations, and narratives continue to affect the rest of the world (Frantzman, 2021). Because the pandemic has become a political issue in the United States, if one candidate favours a certain health solution, the other may oppose it out of politics rather than common wisdom, which has serious consequences (Frantzman, 2021).

A new virus, the coronavirus, is the latest in a long line of diseases that have led to unfair treatment and blame. People in Asia are generally accused of being responsible for the coronavirus, which the U.S. government named the "Chinese Virus" and "Kung Flu" (Clark, 2020). According to Human Rights Watch, this attempt to blame China has stoked "racism and physical attacks against Asians" (Ding & Kananack, 2021).

Government and the public are increasingly aware that scapegoating, which frequently leads to finger-pointing, is counterproductive and only serves to exacerbate current problems by diverting attention away from response efforts and disease containment. Debates about where the Virus emerged and naming specific countries of origin might be unproductive or counterproductive (Baniamin et al., 2020; McNeil, 2010). Investing in the Virus's origin is a waste of time and money, as treating victims and saving lives are more important (Archibold, 2010; Ding & Kananack, 2021).

Ascribing the outbreak in the United States primarily to China is incorrect on both a scientific and a practical level. There is a "contagion of irrationality" being held against many Chinese Americans, despite the fact that many of them have never gone to China. Chinese businesses and residences have been defaced and trashed by the frightened populace, who refuse to dine out or shop at restaurants, and who hurl racial slurs in public (Clark, 2020). Public health officials and the general public are being given conflicting information about how to contain the Virus as a result of this. Politicization can lead to the disease being undermined or dismissed during pandemics. This degree of politicization of pandemics has consequences for racial disparities. A smallpox epidemic during the Civil War killed more black people than whites, and the public was mostly apathetic to the epidemic because it primarily affected black communities; as a result, little medical attention and health response effort was committed to the pandemic (Bavel et al., 2020; Ding & Kananack, 2021).

Cooperation and Compliance

The capabilities of a state and the level of economic inequality among its inhabitants influence its ability to respond effectively to a pandemic like COVID-19. It makes little difference whether the country is a democracy or else (Guillen, 2020). The belief is that greater openness, accountability, and public trust contribute to lower epidemic frequency and fatality, shorter response periods, and higher compliance with public health policy in democracies. Inequality affects the frequency and magnitude of epidemics and people's willingness to cooperate with epidemic containment measures like social distancing and sheltering in place because individuals on the bottom end of the socioeconomic spectrum cannot afford to stay at home. They must work. Powerful governmental and administrative institutions, on the other hand, maybe able to compensate for the majority of deficiencies. The ability of the state protects residents from the start and negative consequences of crises and emergencies, while economic inequality exacerbates them (Guillen, 2020). Countries with a higher state capacity score have fewer of these epidemics because their administrations are more resourceful, regardless of whether the party is in office. And, if they have one, they are likely to have fewer deaths and cases. Guillen (2020) goes on to say that, for the most part, whether you are a democracy or a dictator makes little difference. However, inequality can amplify the consequences of all of this, particularly in terms of the number of people affected (Guillen, 2020).

The COVID-19 catastrophe was compounded by income inequality inside and across countries, resulting in significant geopolitical instability. Economic and social systems frequently aggravate social polarization and endanger national security. In order to establish a more sustainable future while lowering inequality and encouraging shared prosperity, governments must address a number of crucial concerns. While each obstacle is distinct, they are interconnected in such a way that failing to overcome one has a negative impact on the others. As a result, success will necessitate a cross-ministerial, cross-agency executive-level plan (Shannon & Burrowes, 2021). Cities, governments, states, and even local towns have become dysfunctional.

The outbreak exposed a lack of regional and worldwide prevention measures and collaboration. In the context of local interests, collaboration, cooperation, and solidarity have all but vanished within the European Union and the United States of America. There has been a decline in support. Indeed, the vast majority of developing and emerging economies have been left to fend for themselves. When a crisis occurred in the past, both the United States and Western countries sought solutions. For example, at the height of the Cold War, the US and the Soviet Union were locked in a bitter rivalry. This culminated in the 1962 Cuban Missile Crisis, a 13-day standoff provoked by the Soviet Union's decision to station nuclear weapons in Cuba. Even at that time, scientists from the United States and Russia collaborated on at least two vaccines that ultimately saved the world. Prominent US and Russian virologists collaborated to develop vaccines against polio and smallpox, the world's two most prevalent infectious diseases at the time. Between these two countries, science and technology have a long and illustrious history. Scientists from both countries, speaking the same language i.e. language of science. It was a unique chance to progress knowledge and bring about peace in a world that is becoming increasingly frightening, in part because of their own actions (Hilotin, 2020). There is currently no evidence of such behaviour. Both international organizations and governments have shown to be completely ineffectual. It's difficult to understand the lack of global authority in the face of a global pandemic. The Group of Seven, the League of Twenty, and even the BRICS (Brazil, Russia, India, China, and South Africa) have all failed to address the problem (Yenel, 2020).

The traditional international cooperation mechanisms of the existing liberal rules-based order are inadequate in addressing the difficulties of the world governance gap. Existing collaboration structures have been unable to respond adequately to the pandemic. Because of their achievements, the World Bank, the United Nations, the World Trade Organization, the International Monetary Fund, and other international organizations such as the G20 have discussed it. They have not yet effectively created a global united front against the disease (Liao & Tsai, 2019). De-globalization and the rise of populism had already harmed international development cooperation prior to the outbreak of COVID-19. Brexit, Trump's "America First" foreign policy, and the rise of far-right politics are all manifestations of this. The following two aspects are where Xiaoyun et al. (2020) feel the root reasons are located:

To begin, developed countries are concerned about the global economy's strong reliance on developing countries. In terms of the makeup of the global value chain, industrialized countries control a bigger fraction of superior high-value-added capital assets. The withdrawal of industrial sectors from developing countries contributed to increased unemployment in rich countries. Furthermore, the rapid rise of China and other rising countries in recent years, notably in high-tech domains such as 5G (fifth-generation mobile network), has jeopardized numerous established countries' leadership positions in capital-intensive industries. As a result of the "Belt and Road" initiative, China's international influence has grown even further. This has upset wealthier countries with a monopoly position in global value networks.

Second, income redistribution measures in many industrialized countries have failed to reduce economic disparities within their boundaries. For example, at the end of 2017, US President Donald Trump signed the Tax Cuts and Jobs Act (TCJA), which is widely regarded as the country's most significant tax cut in three decades. Capital gains taxes, corporation taxes, Federal Reserve interest rate reductions, and income tax reductions for the middle and lower classes total approximately $1.5 trillion. Tax cuts were meant to boost unemployment, restore economic growth, reduce the country's reliance on foreign markets and capital, and increase consumption and reduce the country's reliance on foreign markets and capital. However, as a result of its tax reform programme, the United States now has the highest fiscal losses among OECD countries. In 2019, the US fiscal deficit reached 960 billion dollars (Xinhua, 2019). Faced with the potential of collapse and public unrest due to the financial crisis, government agencies decided to dissolve organizations, limit foreign support, and reduce multilateral cooperation with international organizations to relieve local economic pressure. In recent years, the United States has withdrawn from over ten international treaties and organizations.

The fast spread of this pandemic in such a short period of time has put pressure on global governance skills, aggravating the sustainable development deficit, which has now transformed into the global governance gap. Global issues like COVID-19 can and should be only be resolved through established international procedures. The global governance players' perspectives on development concerns have altered dramatically since these ideas were introduced. For example, international trade negotiations in the Doha Round have come to a halt, and the United States has withdrawn from the Paris Climate Agreement. Nationalist policies, in fact, will continue to erode the willingness and foundation for international collaboration in the future world order. Only 1% of people in low-income countries have received at least one vaccine dose, compared to 51% in high-income countries, highlighting worldwide vaccine inequities (Solís et al., 2021; Ullah & Nawaz, 2020; Ullah et al., 2021c). The KFF study shows that the disparities by income level and geography of the country have implications for vaccine distribution. Africa has the lowest coverage (2%) while Europe has the highest (40%), followed by the Americas (39%) and the Western Pacific (33%) (KFF, 2021; Solís et al., 2021).

If current vaccination rates continue, low-income nations are unlikely to meet the objectives of 40% by the end of 2021 and 60% by mid-2022 that the WHO

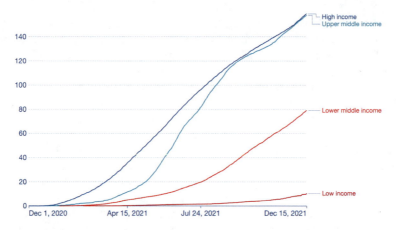

Fig. 3.1 Share of COVID-19 vaccine by income group (*Source* World Bank, 2021)

and World Bank have set out. To achieve 40% coverage by the end of 2021, low-income countries would need to roughly treble their daily vaccination rate. While the Western Pacific, Europe, the Americas, and South-East Asia are on course to fulfil these vaccination targets, Africa's first-dose administration rate will need to be increased eightfold by the end of 2021 to reach 40% (KFF, 2021), which is unlikely (Fig. 3.1).

The pandemic has wreaked devastation on fragile states more than other countries, created widespread unrest, and put international crisis management mechanisms to the test. Its consequences are especially severe for those caught in the crossfire of war if, as appears to be the case, the illness stymies humanitarian relief shipments, hinders peacekeeping operations, and delays or diverts warring parties from launching and sustaining diplomatic efforts. Unscrupulous governments may utilize the outbreak to further their interests in ways that exacerbate internal or international tensions, such as cracking down on domestic opposition or increasing confrontations with rival countries, in order to avoid detection. At the same time, the rest of the world is distracted. COVID-19 has led to strained relations between great powers, with the US blaming China for the outbreak and Beijing seeking allies by delivering aid to affected countries, straining crisis management collaboration even further.

It is unknown when and where the Virus will have the strongest effect and how economic, social, and political elements may interact to cause or exacerbate issues. It is also unclear whether the pandemic's impact on peace and security will be entirely or consistently adverse. Though natural disasters have a history of lowering battles by compelling opposing parties to cooperate or, at the very least, remain mute in order to focus on saving and rebuilding their civilizations. In the aftermath of COVID-19, there are some signs that states are seeking to alleviate political tensions, with the UAE and Kuwait, for example, sending humanitarian aid to Iran, the site of one of the worst first outbreaks outside of China. While the pandemic would most likely exacerbate some global challenges, it may also provide an opportunity to address others. The coming months might be highly perilous, with the focus in the United States and Europe on the domestic impact of COVID-19, while the Virus is projected to spread to impoverished and war-torn countries. COVID-19 primarily impacted states that were able to confront the problem in its early stages, albeit unevenly and at the expense of severe strains on their health systems and economies, such as China, South Korea, and Italy. Until now, fewer instances have been found in countries with weaker healthcare systems, less effective governments, or considerable internal conflict, where an outbreak might be devastating (Abiad et al., 2020; ICG, 2021).

Political Temperature and Responses

It is comprehensible that politicians would like not to have to make decisions about which candidates to support because doing so comes with political risks, such as alienating individuals who are left out or having to deal with the aftermath of the choices are made incorrectly. Interestingly, the most politically expedient path of action is not always the most economically advantageous course of action. When it comes to businesses like restaurants and artisan shops on the street, the public has a strong desire to support them even when they open and close on a regular basis. If public funds are to be used to support existing businesses, they should not be utilized to pay rent, salaries, or interest on idle assets. Instead, it may be better to reduce public assistance. By renegotiating leases and bank loans, some businesses may be able to stay afloat. Others, on the other hand, may not be able to. Losing bartenders should be compensated with unemployment compensation, but the businesses where they worked should be shut down. If demand shifts, they can reopen, rehire personnel, or rebrand as e-sports parlours. More important is protecting the worker in the event of a lockdown than protecting the job (Alvarez et al., 2020; Rajan, 2021).

While the current coronavirus pandemic has sparked heated rhetoric and retaliatory recriminations between the USA and China, what has been happening beyond China's eastern and southern borders for several months is equally significant. At a time when the Chinese Communist Party boasts of its generous approach to COVID-19, the number of incidents between China and its neighbours has soared (Denmark et al., 2020). Beijing has increased tensions, investigated responses, and determined how much it can get away with using its naval and paramilitary forces, as well as more sophisticated media operations. The epidemic has exacerbated pre-existing inter-state political tensions. COVID-19, for example, has visibly aggravated tensions between India and Pakistan over Kashmir and Afghanistan. While both countries are fighting the pandemic, we may witness more entrenchment of the armed status quo and domestic initiatives revealing the Indian government's vulnerability to the pandemic. Indian nationalist tactics are being used successfully to divert public attention away from the COVID-19 situation (Staniland, 2020).

As a result of many nations downplaying or simply rejecting the situation, international guidance to address the COVID-19 pandemic turned insufficient. Even when the World Health Organization designated COVID-19 a pandemic, several of the world's most powerful countries downplayed the danger. Because of their geographical location, many leaders believed they could combat the Virus, and scientists tried to persuade them otherwise. As the number of cases and deaths grew, numerous nations remained skeptical about the Virus's lethality and contagiousness. Ignorance isn't always comfortable; it can be deadly. Wild claims and downright misleading and false news are proliferating in some countries while facts are buried, inciting fear and rendering preventive actions useless. Disagreements over how to confine and prevent the patient from spreading have hampered the task of containing and stopping it from spreading. Disinformation operations on social media compound the problem and add to the confusion (Yenel, 2020).

Some political leaders in South Asia were heard to say that they were stronger than the COVID-19. This was, in fact, to threaten the opposition parties. Countries with supranational governance institutions, such as the European Union, have struggled over new policies. Amid hurdles during the negotiations, EU members finally agreed on an economic rescue plan in July 2020, despite protests from "frugal" countries over the cost of such proposals (Lee, 2020). However, conflicts over seasonal migrant labour have escalated tensions inside the EU, for example, in Belarus and the EU. Certain businesses, particularly farmers, have advocated for hiring foreign employees, while populist leaders have advocated for harsher immigration policies (Carroll, 2020).

China's economic expansion and determined actions in regions like the South China Sea have put the US's power to the test. The EU's perils, such as Brexit and the growth of non-liberal governments on the periphery, are also putting liberal democracy to the test. All three regions are at the epicentre of the worldwide public health disaster. The Virus originated in China, but the vast majority of fatalities occurred in the United States and Western Europe (as of May 2020). China's efforts to deny that it is not the source of the Virus's emergence and India and the United States' efforts to establish that China purposefully spread the Virus have pushed the world into another cold war-like situation. Given that the public healthcare problem has only been in place for a few weeks, analysing the long-term repercussions of great power rivalry would be premature. We may, however, identify the circumstances that will influence its outcome. Relationships are strained, and the crisis has intensified the incentive to confront rather than cooperate. Despite widespread unemployment and criticism of his management, President Trump was escalating his pressure on China as the November election nears. Furthermore, the President characterized the illness as a "Chinese virus," implying that it was created in a government lab. His administration was debating whether to allow lawsuits against Chinese officials to be filed in the US. On the other hand, the Chinese leadership may be concerned that the end of decades of economic expansion will erode its domestic credibility. The logical path to regaining credibility appears to be through nationalism. Indeed, some Chinese officials had already chastised the US, accusing it of spreading the Virus in the country. By participating in and leading global organizations, alliances, bilateral ties, and soft power, modern great powers fight for the favour of surrounding countries. Of course, under President Trump, the United States has reduced its total foreign responsibilities (Eiran, 2020).

The pandemic presents a variety of new threats to state stability. COVID-19 has enabled armed opposition organizations to scale up their attacks and, in some instances, target authority opponents. Political violence, domestic military action, and state failure are all potential sites of escalation. Rebel organizations and other violent actors have used these chances to consolidate authority, attain political goals, and increase their capacity to administer and enforce rules. Armed organizations operating along Colombia's southwest coast, for example, have publicly said that curfew offender will be considered as "military objectives" (Janetsky & Faiola, 2020; Weiss, 2020).

As the COVID-19 Virus spreads fast throughout Sub-Saharan Africa (SSA), the region faces a political crisis as well as health and economic catastrophe. After a brief period in which infection rates were low and confined in only a few countries, media and governments in many of the region's states in SSA were reluctant to recognize the threat. While most of the Global South was initially immune to the COVID-19 pandemic that ravaged China, it then swiftly spread across Europe and the United States due to its geographic location. That grace period was over. Several Sub-Saharan African governments have found themselves in the midst of a political crisis as a result of the COVID-19 outbreak and hence the tardy and inconsistent reaction to it were evident (Devermont & Olander, 2020).

The Virus's rapid spread has shifted media narratives drastically. When it came to African media coverage of the expanding COVID-19 story, it had to fight with stories on South African cooking recipes on News24, Kenyan domestic political disputes on Daily Nation, and Nigerian criticism of President Buhari's leadership on Premium Times to get any traction. Things, on the other hand, have suddenly changed. The story of COVID-19 has spread well beyond the health section of a news website. Kenya, South Africa and Nigeria, among many other countries, are directly affected by this story (Devermont & Olander, 2020).

Democracy in Southeast Asia has deteriorated, notwithstanding the political stagnation. A substantial COVID-19 epidemic has now occurred in the region following the region's escape from the 2020 pandemic. Personal destruction and economic devastation accompany an anti-political uprising brought on by the new wave (Kurlantzick, 2021a, 2021b). South and Southeast Asia were at the forefront of a worldwide democratization movement from the late 1980s to the early 2000s. Political reforms were made in Thailand, Indonesia, the Philippines, East Timor, and Cambodia; however, Cambodia, Malaysia, and Myanmar did not. It has been a rough few years for the region's political fortunes, as the region has fallen into line with the general decline in democracy around the world since the late 2000s. In any case, the pandemic is raising the resentment of the region's leaders, which could lead to a return to democratic growth (Kurlantzick, 2021a, 2021b).

South Asian countries are reeling from a new and devastating epidemic of COVID-19. More than half of all new infections in the world are occurring in this region, which is home to more than two billion people. More than three cases are reported every second. Death rates are also rising. Three more people in the area lose their lives to the disease every minute (Unicef, 2021). For decades, South Asia has been plagued by poor governance systems and healthcare services that reach the most vulnerable populations. India and Pakistan, the region's two most powerful countries, stand in the way of resolving these challenges. South Asian politics have also been complicated by foreign factors such as Cold War bloc politics, the war on terrorism, and, more recently, the rising Sino-US competition. Hence, we see the Prime Minister, ministers, and the Presidents go overseas for their own treatment (Ullah & Huque, 2019). There were three South Asian Association for Regional Cooperation (SAARC) countries that were severely afflicted by avian flu: Afghanistan, Bangladesh, and Pakistan. The second-highest daily average of COVID-19 instances in the world was recorded in India. On the other hand, a second wave of the Virus is sweeping over Sri Lanka, where the infection was first confined. Increased infection rates are forcing the governments of Bangladesh, Nepal and Pakistan to adopt more drastic measures to stop the spread of the Virus.

Two major barriers have hindered the response to the pandemic in the region. First, many of the restrictions imposed are unworkable due to a lack of basic healthcare and sanitation services in the affected areas concerned. The United Nations Human Development Report ranks Sri Lanka 72nd out of 72 countries in the region with a score of 0.782. People in the country who are suspected of having COVID-19 have had an extraordinarily high percentage of recovery up until this point. People have died in their homes or on the way to the nearest hospital in other sections of the region (Senaratne, 2020). Over two decades of border disputes in South Asia, the forced migration of Burmese Muslims to Bangladesh, the rise of the Taliban in Afghanistan, and a significant outflow of professionals and educated women exiting the country in 2021 all demonstrate how volatile and difficult to predict this region is. Interstate "water wars" may become a reality as a result of climate change (Bhalla, 2012). Despite an increase in threats in South Asia, interstate violence remains a distinct possibility.

Africa

The levels of preparedness of the governments of the region compounded the disparity in their responses. The majority of African governments implemented some kind of lockdown during the early phases of the pandemic. However, in countries that responded by proclaiming a state of emergency, others faced severe challenges due to a lack of proper safety net resources and faced significant hurdles in maintaining their social isolation. Only a few of these countries, including South Africa, were able to completely flatten the curve before it reopened.

Light social distance methods were used in several countries because they were concerned about the cost lockdown may cause. Instead, they relied on personal hygiene and self-preservation, making "life for livelihood" compromises. The youth of the region were hit hard by COVID-19 lockdown. Although the health services are poor, current figures show that the region reduced the death rate from infection. Overall, the COVID-19 mortality risk is predicted to be 2.3%, compared to 2.4% globally (Mutapi, 2021).

Due to a containment policy, African economies have been severely impacted by domestic activities being suspended. Global response to the pandemic, which included border restrictions (which hurt trade and tourism), the fall of global demand (for oil, for example, hurt African oil producers), and supply chain disruptions, may have caused the most serious loss (Ndulu, 2020). This means that Sub-Saharan Africa is expected to see its first downturn in 25 years in 2021 and 2022. Globally, the International Monetary Fund (IMF) predicted that GDP in the region would fall by 3.2% in 2020 before increasing by 3.4% the following year. Nigeria and South Africa, the two largest economies in the region, have been the most influential by the end of 2020 (with 5.4 and 8% contractions, respectively). The region's recession would be substantially less severe, at –0.6%, and it would recover faster, with 3.8% growth in 2021. About 14 out of 45 countries can overcome a recession, although growth will be much slower than in 2019 (Ndulu, 2020).

An estimated 85.8% of Africans are employed in the informal sector (ILO, 2020a). Those in lower-income brackets were more likely to be affected by the pandemic. There has been a 9.1% increase in extreme poverty in Sub-Saharan Africa since COVID-19, with lockdowns accounting for 65% of the increase. Reports predict that 3.6% of the region's population, including 3.9 million children under the age of five, are at risk from acute food insecurity (Ndulu, 2020). Hence, recovery is not just about regaining lost ground; rather it is also about addressing the distributional effects and bringing those who have slipped below the poverty line.

Latin America

In the wake of COVID-19, the global economy is in shambles, and emerging economies are no exception. After a brief pause, this shock quickly spread over Asia and the rest of the world, with Latin America particularly hard hit. As a result of the delta variant's complexity and rapid transmissibility within the region, Latin America continues to have considerably more cases of infection than any other region, even after the latest outbreak in Asia (García-Herrero, 2021). As a result of a faster transmission of the Virus, a more significant economic impact, and more restrictive policy responses, Latin America falls short of policy stimulus. According to the IMF's policy tracker, Japan has initiated a stimulus programme totalling 15.6% of GDP, Singapore 16.3%, Brazil 8.3%, and Mexico 0.7% (García-Herrero, 2021).

There is no doubt that Latin America was hit harder than the rest of the world, and the rebuilding process was slower as a result. Debt dynamics have worsened in Latin American countries, and dollar financing has become increasingly difficult to get. The Regional Reserve Fund for Latin America (FLAR) regional insurance plan is still in its infancy in the region, which has much less foreign exchange reserves available for self-insurance (García-Herrero, 2021). The high fatality rates in the region have been attributed to two structural reasons. The first one, economic disparity and that a large informal sector has been a part of Latin American history for a long time. Individuals may or may not have abided by tight quarantine measures that were enforced by several nations during the pandemic. More than a few low-income people, particularly those involved in informal work, were forced to leave their houses in order to make ends meet. At the same time, much of Latin America's housing has been self-built in informal settlements. Many people live in close proximity, making the transmission of viruses easy, which may have sped up the spread of the Virus in some areas. The second structural challenge is that health services around the region still fall short of the personnel and technical resources they need to tackle the pandemic successfully. The pandemic is predicted to be more lethal in Latin America because of a lack of oxygen supplies, restricted vaccine supplies, and sluggish vaccination rollouts (Holland, 2021). US ex-President Donald Trump's example greatly influenced the response of other regional leaders. Brazilian President Jair Bolsonaro, who looked forward to Trump and rejected the gravity of the threat of the pandemic in the same fashion, left local governors and mayors to implement their own measures and counter public message that lowered the threat. Bolsonaro also showed a reluctance to enact lockdowns or mask policies (Holland, 2021).

There are two methods to approach this topic. In the first instance, we saw a convergence of two occurrences in the region, both of which were exacerbated by the epidemic. After the commodities boom, Latin America was able to adopt new social programmes amid a period of fast expansion and economic advancement (Fernandez & Machado, 2021). There was an increase in school and college enrollment as a result of the boom. People had high hopes for social mobility as a result. Growth slowed, and aspirations for upward mobility faded as the commodities boom ended in 2013. The pandemic has crushed even people's aspirations: children are dropping out of school, people are getting unemployed, social programmes are undercrowded, and many people believe social mobility is now impossible. As the virus spread, many people began to assume their governments had abandoned them. As a result of the commodities boom in Latin America, a massive corruption scandal and a massive misuse of resources occurred (Holland, 2021). And that corruption scandals have a negative impact on the public's faith in their governments.

It's also possible to look at the impact of government performance on regional politics during the outbreak, which is much less apparent. However, some politicians have emerged relatively unscathed from the disastrous reaction to the pandemic. Until recently, for example, Bolsonaro was widely supported in Brazil despite the country's rising death toll. One of the reasons for this is that he was also significantly involved in transferring money to help people survive the outbreak (Weiffen, 2020). When it comes to the Ebola epidemic, Mexico's Andrés Manuel López Obrador won the June midterm elections. Still, he did not develop an adequate public health response or establish social programmes for the poor. For example, countries like Chile and Peru followed public health advice to the letter, although their presidents ' popularity and trust in the government didn't rise. According to what we believe to be an underlying narrative of social malaise and distrust of government, the actions done by governments during the epidemic have had little impact (Holland, 2021; Weiffen, 2020).

Asia

Despite the global scope of the COVID-19 and its associated economic challenges, both crises have profound local consequences. Both crises necessitate swift and perfect policy responses. On the other hand, global concerns necessitate global cooperation and coordination, and individual countries cannot accomplish this on their own. The restricted movement became more frequent as the outbreak developed into a true worldwide pandemic in February and March 2020. Several Asian countries quickly enacted travel restrictions as well. Lockdowns have become normal throughout Europe and portions of the United States, where infection rates were significantly higher than in Asia. There is widespread anxiety about what restrictions may still be imposed, how they would affect viral containment, and when they would be repealed.

The Migration Domain

Is the migration landscape going to reshape? The COVID-19 pandemic has exacerbated international migrants' pre-existing fears. As a result of the financial crisis, numerous firms were compelled to lay off workers, causing the outbreak to largely affect temporary economic migrants. While governments have devised economic policies to assist enterprises, temporary migrants are typically excluded from these programmes (Staynor, 2020). Several countries are also considering changing their migration policy and drastically changing their approach to asylum requests. For example, limiting face-to-face interviews, erecting additional physical walls, or requiring asylum seekers to bring their own black or blue ink pens. Internal migration is not spared too. Internal migrants also face impositions and restrictions in terms of mobility (Bonotti & Zech, 2021; Nott, 2020).

Women and girls around the world have lesser rights and freedoms than men and boys, especially when it comes to basic matters like their bodies and fate (Beltramo et al., 2021). Eighteen countries allow husbands to legally forbid their wives from working; 39 countries do not treat daughters and sons equally when it comes to inheriting; and 49 countries lack legislation to protect women from domestic abuse (UN SDG, 2021). More than a year after the COVID-19 outbreak, data demonstrate that previously existing disparities are widening, showing vulnerabilities in the social, political and economic systems of women and girls all around the world.

Data Especially for marginalized and poor women, women shoulder a disproportionately greater amount of household duties (such as child care) than males (Beltramo et al., 2021).

There is an increased risk of transmission of the Virus among female refugees due to poor living conditions as well as poor sanitation and medical care. These people are more vulnerable to infection (Crawley, 2021), who live in congested and unclean surroundings than any group of population. Because of their shaky financial standing, they are frequently left out of humanitarian efforts to fight poverty and famine. Despite the fact that women are more likely to spend extended periods of time away from work to care for their children, men are freer to engage in non-work activities. The immediate impact of health crises combines with financial and food poverty due to the delay in delivering humanitarian help, undermining migrants' resilience and ability to cope in the long term. Countries with a history of conflict or that have become refugees have a more challenging time doing business as a whole (Rahmadhani et al., 2021; UNHCR, 2017).

There is a growing sense of exclusion and exceptionalism among refugees as a result of protective policies, as well as a growing sense of material insecurity. As an alternative, COVID-19 provides the Global South with an excuse to tighten border controls. At an alarming pace, refugees are being denied international safeguards to which they are entitled. Partisan politicians who stand to gain financially from the epidemic are using them as scapegoats (along with refugees in general) (Ullah, 2014). Several governments have implemented controversial laws that further restrict refugee access to legitimize and rationalize refugee marginalization. Instead of changing the course of refugee protection history, COVID-19 appears to accelerate it. Following the COVID-19 crisis, numerous Asian nations have imposed travel restrictions and lockdown measures that resulted in massive job losses and limited mobilization of migrant workers, leading to labour rights abuses and poor health and community safety (Ullah, Haji-Othman, & Daud, 2021). The policies restricting women and undocumented migrant workers, the contracts that are insufficient, and the devaluation of domestic work make them particularly susceptible (UN Women, 2020).

Many jobs have been lost, and those who face labour rights breaches such as increased working hours and inadequate COVID-19 protection measures because of the temporary halt in operations (OECD, 2020a). Families in countries like Nepal and Myanmar, where remittances are heavily relied upon, are put at risk of poverty when migrant workers are forced to return home. The number of returnees is increasing day by day, resulting in a decline in the remittances flow. This leads to severe difficulty for millions of families to escape poverty, improve their living standards in the areas of education and health, and obtain land, as well as pay off their debts (Poudel & Subedi, 2020). Aside from the suspension of shelter applications, refugees have faced discrimination. Several Arab states and the European Union have imposed discriminatory limitations on Syrian refugees (Ullah, 2018). Governments are mainly lying when they claim that these different measures are vital for public health (Table 3.1).

Table 3.1 Estimated reduction in global and regional remittances flow

	Amount ($ million)	% of baseline
World	56,603–108,617	9.7–18.3
Developing Asia	31,016–53,460	11.6–20.0
Central Asia	2,228–3,366	15.7–23.8
East Asia	4,209–9,546	5.8–13.1
Southeast Asia	6,187–11,660	9.9–18.6
South Asia	18,276–28,621	15.8–24.7
The Pacific	116–267	5.7–13.2
United States	226–482	3.5–7.4
Europe	8,071–17,889	6.5–16.4
Rest of the world	18,290–36,786	9.3–18.8

Source Takenaka et al. (2020)

The Public Health

Over the previous several decades, a growing amount of literature has revealed how market forces have increasingly influenced current healthcare research, financing, and delivery (De Vogli, 2011; Keshavjee & Farmer, 2014). Throughout the early 1980s, countries in the Global South, particularly in Latin America and Africa, faced a growing debt crisis, which necessitated significant changes in economic and public health policies as heavily indebted countries were forced to make a variety of "structural adjustments" in order to secure loans from international financial institutions (Kentikelenis et al., 2016). While the trend of global health governance toward market-led approaches over the last several decades has been thoroughly researched (Benatar et al., 2018), fewer studies have examined the relationship between this movement and the rise of digital health technologies. Wamsley and Chin-Yee suggest that the spread of digital technology in healthcare occurred in concert with the market euphoria and techno-optimism associated with the late 1990s and early 2000s New Economy, rather than as a result of politically neutral technological efficiency efforts. Along with a series of geopolitical, economic, and public health crises, technology solutions to "new" and "unprecedented" problems have received growing political and widespread attention (Wamsley & Chin-Yee, 2021).

States have responded differently to the COVID-19 epidemic in different conditions. While few countries have successfully contained the Virus's spread, the fragmentation of public health responses in liberal capitalist countries has been particularly pronounced, with persistent challenges in reducing community transmission, managing hospital capacity, mobilizing centralized contact tracing, increasing PPE provision, and protecting vulnerable populations (Mellish et al., 2020). Within the market-led healthcare system in the United States, for example, a fragmented federal response that devolved public health authority to state and local governments (Haffajee & Mello, 2020) and a reluctance to enforce centralized public health measures to temporarily halt market activity both contributed to the COVID-19 devastation (Wamsley & Chin-Yee, 2021).

When applied to digital health technology, this lens illustrates how digitalization corresponded with significant changes in global health governance that favoured market-based methods. Perceived crises reinforced techno-solutionist discourses and expedited the integration of private-sector technologies into global public health systems (OECD, 2020b). While the effectiveness of technological responses to the COVID-19 pandemic has varied across global contexts and remains unknown, rapid adoption of digital health technologies has frequently displaced or reduced the need for large-scale public health interventions, potentially exacerbating underlying social and health inequalities (Wamsley & Chin-Yee, 2021).

To combat COVID-19, health care facilities must have enough water, sanitation, hygiene, and clinical waste management systems, as well as adequate cleaning. The WHO and UNICEF baseline study from 2019 states that an estimated 896 million people use health services without access to water, and 1.5 billion people use facilities without access to sanitation (Human Rights Watch, 2020; UnWater, 2019). The World Health Organization (WHO) sent contradictory messages depending on the information provided by countries rather than technical evidence, leading to the organization being viewed as politically oriented and incapable of giving vital advice and assistance. This is demonstrated by their swift delivery of 300 kits to northwest Syria, which is home to about four million civilians and displaced people. The fractured and chaotic image of nations closing borders and hospitals overwhelmed by insufficient supplies calls into question the viability and effectiveness of international and regional institutions, increasing nationalism and xenophobia. This left a void, which China is now filling in to appease countries upset by the economic neglect from the west (Kahf, 2020). The public health issue is influencing domestic political tensions in a variety of ways. Certain politicians, for example, utilized the outbreak to their political advantage during the EU-UK post-Brexit negotiations (Leonard, 2020). Politicians have periodically questioned experts' authority, undermining citizens' trust in evidence-based reasoning (Olorunnipa, 2020). In order to further their ideas, they regularly mischaracterized or usurped scientific expertise on topics—for example, mask-wearing (Aratani, 2020). Political differences have fostered and intensified disputes about the pandemic in several countries, resulting in clashes between national and regional political authorities. Calls for unification and systemic reform, on the other hand, have occasionally served to bridge ideological and political divides (Jiang et al., 2020). Furthermore, the outbreak raises a more critical political question: should healthcare be considered primarily a "public benefit" or a "private choice?"

Gender has a critical implication for health care services. In numerous countries, healthcare providers discriminate against lesbians, gay men, and transgender people. Among other places, Human Rights Watch (2020) has documented discrimination based on gender or sexual orientation in health care in the United States and Russia, in Japan as well as Tanzania, Indonesia, Bangladesh and Lebanon. Due to this discrimination, LGBTs may have a harder time getting tested for HIV and treated, or receiving care for other chronic diseases, increasing their risk of serious illness or death from COVID-19 (Human Rights Watch, 2020). Things like typhoid or smallpox are relegated to the realm of horror stories. The annual death toll from non-communicable diseases like heart disease and cancer has risen to 71%. Mental diseases often necessitate individual rather than collective healthcare decisions. The health of any community, rich or poor, is put in jeopardy when confronted with an epidemic like COVID-19 that necessitates a coordinated response. To contain the outbreak, a systemic reaction is needed, which puts individual risks and costs on hold. The outbreak of the COVID-19 Virus has also drawn attention to healthcare policy on a global scale, especially when governments' ability to deliver certain services is being curtailed by tightening budgets. As a result of the coronavirus epidemic, some countries, most notably Europe, where public health care is an important part of the social compact but has been constrained by budgetary constraints, should reassess their fiscal priorities. According to French President Emmanuel Macron, it is important to maintain and prioritize medical care as a public benefit (Dauba-Pantanacce, 2020).

During the COVID-19 pandemic, the Human Rights Council (HRC) expressed grave concern about new policies blocking and punishing the free flow of information. People have died as a result of governments lying, concealing facts, detaining journalists, failing to notify the public about the magnitude of the threat, and criminalizing individuals under the pretence of spreading false information. People have suffered because some governments would prefer to avoid criticism than allow people to share information, learn about the outbreak, and understand what officials are or are not doing to protect them. Many countries (including Belarus, Cambodia, China, Iran, Egypt, India, Myanmar, Bangladesh, and Turkey) have utilized the COVID epidemic to stifle free expression in contravention of their human rights commitments. The UN hence calls on governments around the world to take measures to defend and promote free speech during the COVID-19 pandemic, which several countries have used to crack down on journalists and suppress critics. This has hampered communication about the roots of the disease and eroded public faith in government efforts.

The ongoing conflict between Asia's two most considerable growing powers (China and India) may benefit the countries. Though the rising competitiveness in health diplomacy presents a variety of issues. While China and India pursue different goals and techniques, they both operate in the same arena. Their health policy may overlap with other sectors, increasing their competitiveness, if not aggressiveness. External powers have an impact on the dynamics between the two countries as well. The United States, Japan, and Australia joined forces with India at the recent Quad Summit to challenge China's growing influence. If rivalry gets so fierce that smaller countries are forced to pick sides, the Indo-Pacific region would face new challenges (Yang et al., 2021). The leaders of Australia, the United Kingdom, and the United States (AUKUS) later announced the formation of a new trilateral military collaboration. India has been excluded from AUKUS, however. These three Anglo-American countries plan to cooperate in areas such as artificial intelligence, cybersecurity, long-range attack, quantum computing, and subsea technologies (Korybko, 2021).

Disparity

Inequality continues to grow. Despite the economic costs of the COVID-19 pandemic, more than five million people globally became millionaires in 2020. Despite the fact that many impoverished people have become poorer, Credit Suisse estimates indicate that worldwide millionaires have climbed by 5.2–56.1 million. By 2020, more than 1% of the world's population became millionaires, and their fortunes were helped by rising stock markets and home values (BBC, 2020).

According to many researches, decreased interest rates on loans and government assistance have resulted in a "massive transfer" of wealth from the public to private sectors. As a result, household savings surged, inflating household financial assets and deflationary pressures to levels not seen since the Great Depression. By 2020, the number of people with investable assets over $30 million will have climbed by a staggering 24%, the highest rate since 2003 (Ullah & Huque, 2019).

Between $6.1 trillion and $9.1 trillion, or 7.1–10.5% of global GDP will be lost, according to the ADB's (2021) estimate. The impact on developing Asian countries is expected to be between $1.3 trillion and $2.0 trillion, or 5.7–8.5% of developing Asia's GDP, which is around 22% of the worldwide loss (Sawada & Sumulong, 2021). Economic losses of 5.5–8.7% in 2020 and 3.6–6.3% for 2021 are projected by the ADB's most current MRIOT-based impact estimate, which was released in December 2020. Losses in emerging Asia in 2020 and 2021 are comparable to regional GDP losses that range from 6.0 to 9.5% (Abiad et al., 2020c).

Economic disparities between the rich and poor can be worsened by a variety of factors (Zhuang, 2020). While all wage earners would be affected, most low-skilled workers will bear the brunt of the impact. Due to the epidemic, jobs have become skill-biased, i.e. routine and manual employment have become increasingly vulnerable to automation. As a second factor, the pandemic will disproportionately affect poor and vulnerable groups such as MSMEs, women, the elderly, and those employed in labour-intensive and service sectors, such as nursing homes. As a result of the economic contractions, labour and capital owners alike are likely to suffer. However, the latter, who are often wealthier and more involved in hard-hit service sectors, are more likely to be affected than the former. Even though poor regions typically lack the capacity to execute containment measures and offer proper healthcare, the pandemic could aggravate the regional income gap, resulting in a slower recovery after the epidemic (Sawada & Sumulong, 2021).

The pandemic has wrecked devastation on people's lives in every country and region. It will significantly negatively impact global economic growth around 2021 and beyond, something that has not happened in nearly a century. The COVID-19 outbreak remains a deeply personal and individual experience, as well as a once-in-a-generation worldwide phenomenon with far-reaching implications. The Virus is expected to have a negative impact on the global economy of −3.4 to −7.6% in 2020, before rebounding to 4.2–5.6% in 2021. Global trade is anticipated to fall by 5.3% in 2020 but to rise by 8.0% in 2021 (IMF, 2021). According to mainstream estimates, the economic downturn in 2020 would be milder than expected, owing

Disparity

in part to fiscal and monetary policies undertaken by governments in 2020. The severity of the health crisis and its influence on the global economy has placed doubt on economic growth estimates, which had previously expected a decrease in economic growth followed by a rebound in the second and third quarters of 2020 (CRS, 2021). The epidemic ravaged the aviation industry first, followed by tourism, athletics, and cultural activities. Closed borders hampered commerce in almost every economic area; a chain reaction resulted in a downward spiral. Unemployment has risen across the board. Economic revival will necessitate the government playing a larger role. These operations, however, will necessitate the involvement of foreign financial institutions (Yenel, 2020).

The outbreak of COVID-19 has destruction on the global economy, creating a global recession. Traditional strategies such as restricting economic activity flow, compressing markets, and shutting down the financial services distribution network have all been deployed to gain time for anti-pandemic measures. Some governments have provided unprecedented levels of indirect support to businesses and individuals in the form of money, investment, tax breaks, and commodities distribution. However, this amount of support has come at the expense of the government's debt. The World Bank predicts a 4% increase in global output in 2021, assuming universal COVID-19 vaccination efficacy and government policies and programmes that encourage private sector growth while reducing public sector debt (Shannon & Burrowes, 2021). As many industrialized economies begin to recover, central banks and governments are weighing the implications of reducing monetary and fiscal support in light of projected inflationary pressures and the possibility of slowing the speed of recovery. These worries are amplified by the introduction of new disease types and the spread of epidemic hotspots. The top industrialized economies will account for 60% of global economic growth (Vela, 2020) until at least 2024, meaning lower individual and national financial well-being than before the epidemic.

In contrast to the coordinated prediction of a global economic recession in the first half of 2020, the global economy has demonstrated evidence of a two-track recovery that began in the fall of 2020. It is distinguished by a shaky recovery in affluent countries and a slower recovery in emerging economies. Globally, developed countries have raised immunization rates, improving the chances of economic recovery in 2021, and, as a result, the global economy as a whole—the new COVID-19 variant has witnessed a surge in patients in key emerging economies. Furthermore, vaccine tolerance among certain sectors of the population in developed economies calls into question the short-term speed and vigour of economic advancement. Lockdowns and curfews have been called for across Europe, the United States, Russia, Brazil, Japan, India, and Africa due to the rise of hazardous diseases. It has the ability to stymie or postpone long-term economic growth until mid-to late-2021. Certain industries and demographic groups have borne a disproportionate part of the epidemic's economic effects. As a result of chronically high unemployment levels not seen since the 1930s economic depression, prolonged labour disruption is possible. Workers reassess their career choices and work patterns in specific circumstances, signalling a post-pandemic economy with more diverse labour arrangements and a changing metropolitan environment (CRS, 2021).

Throughout the coronavirus outbreak, European governments displayed an exceptional willingness to raise spending by covering the wages of furloughed workers. Furthermore, the European Commission suspended EU budgetary standards, allowing countries to pause vital parts of their economy. Even the most financially conservative member countries, such as Austria and the Netherlands, have proposed substantial stimulus measures. Perhaps most importantly, the German government has promptly abandoned, if temporarily, the so-called "black zero" goal of balanced budgets that has characterized the country's economic approach in recent years (Arce et al., 2021; Bergsen et al., 2020). According to the COVID-19 Summit Proclamation, the G20 is infusing about $5 trillion into the global economy to address the pandemic's social, financial, and economic implications. When major economies, including Europe, the United States, and even Japan, enter a phase of negative interest rates in response to the crisis, their ultra-easy fiscal policies may result in competitive devaluation.

In terms of economic policy, the 2008 global financial crisis and the struggling European economy of 2010 burst one after the other, leaving industrialized countries' public debt levels virtually unaltered. The stimulus spending measures to battle the epidemic may further aggravate the financial crisis. To shield the economy from the effects of the epidemic, the US Federal Reserve cut lending rates to zero (twice) and launched a quantitative easing programme. However, the extremely stringent restrictions failed to prevent the US stock market from collapsing four times in ten days in March (2021), underlining the country's significant structural flaws, which are expected to lead to the formation of systemic hazards throughout the economy. Globalization will continue in the post-pandemic world, but at a slower pace and with a different worldview. By far, global trade and investment will decline in size. The World Trade Organization predicts a drop in global trade of between 13 and 32% in 2021. However, this will ultimately be determined by the market economy's rationality and the profit-driven character of capital (ADB, 2020; WTO, 2020a). According to Eiran (2020), while the COVID-19 health concern in Africa appears to be minor, the economic impact on the region is enormous. The African Development Bank (AfDB) has forecast a $500 billion economic loss, which is being investigated. Economists worry that countries in Africa's early lockdown of their sectors and trade restrictions, frightened of the Virus's rapid spread, will have a massive financial impact. The extraction of oil and natural gas and tourism are more vulnerable sectors of the continent's economy. Unlike the United States and other wealthy countries, the region lacks the financial wherewithal to infuse trillions of dollars into its economy. According to AfDB President Akinwumi Adesina, African countries now have access to a $10 billion bank loan. According to the World Bank (2020), Sub-Saharan Africa's economic growth would plummet from 2.4% in 2019 to −2.1 and −5.1% in 2020. The World Bank's foreboding predictions go even farther, forecasting that Sub-Saharan Africa would see its first recession in 25 years.

Female empowerment, which can take many forms, is crucial for achieving gender equality. They can make educational and culinary decisions for their children, in addition to empowering them to make key life decisions for themselves, such as leaving an abusive environment and relationship. As demonstrated by earlier feminist movements, women's involvement may attract attention to the significance of developing more egalitarian and caring workplaces and working conditions for all. For a variety of reasons, the informal sector of any economy employs millions of people, most of whom are women. Today, construction, transportation, small and medium-sized enterprises, domestic and care jobs, and the gig economy employ these workers. They usually travel to places where this kind of labour is available. While migrant women are less likely to be primary breadwinners, they often accompany their partners or families to cities, where they work in informal jobs or care for their homes and children. As a result of random lockdowns and closures in many countries, migrant workers have been compelled to return to their homes, which are mostly rural (Rahmadhani et al., 2021). They experienced challenges along the road.

Self-employed women and participating family workers, such as unpaid family workers in family businesses, agriculture, or the local household sector, are examples of vulnerable workers. Employment vulnerability is expressed as a proportion of total paid and self-employed employment. Women in Asian countries are significantly more likely to find a precarious jobs. Women in this sector are more likely to work in family-owned firms (most typically agricultural), with poor development, irregular employment, and a lack of social security and safety nets. A high incidence of susceptible employment may also suggest a sizable rural economy with slow, formal economic growth (World Bank, 2020).

Gender

In terms of economic status, well-being, safety, and housing and educational settings, women in poverty are one of the groups most touched by the current COVID-19 problem. Individuals suffer considerable inequalities in "normal" times; however, the COVID-19 crisis exacerbates these inequalities and acts as a magnifying glass, focusing light on their specific problems (Equinet, 2021). Women in poverty endure intersectional bias because of their gender and financial status. Individuals' experiences with inequality and prejudice, on the other hand, are typically three-dimensional, as they are linked to other criteria such as their ethnicity, age, or handicap. Women in poverty are diverse; they include Roma women, Muslim women, Black women, Asian women, migrant women, trans women, older women, women with disabilities, single mothers, and others.

Women were the majority in most countries in frontline sectors (supermarket cashiers, teachers, health workers, care workers, and so on), where they faced stress and anxiety due to COVID-19 potential exposure, a lack of prevention measures, and uncertainties, in addition to their generally precarious working conditions. Self-isolation policies failed to examine the unstable conditions of the victims of domestic violence, the impact of suspending in-person services for those with impairments, the impacts of school closures on gender dynamics, or the ramifications of single-parent families, to mention a few instances. Women in poverty have unequal access to technology and the internet, increasing their risk of isolation—especially during lockdowns in many countries—and limiting their capacity to express their ideas. All of this can contribute to greater tension, anxiety, lower levels of life satisfaction, and less free time for poor women (Qin et al., 2020; Equinet, 2021).

In order to better understand the current vulnerabilities and new threats posed by the COVID-19 situation for women in poverty, a task force from the Working Group on Gender Equality issued a discussion paper outlining the experiences of disadvantaged women (Equinet, 2021). 'Women in Poverty: Breaking the Cycle,' the resulting publication, includes "voices from the field" from organizations that work directly with victims of gender discrimination, gender-based violence, and abuse, many of whom are also affected by poverty and social exclusion. The study represents the many lived experiences of disadvantaged women. Rather than offering solutions and ideas, it raises concerns about the critical stages and long-term solutions needed to better the status of all women living in poverty.

There are some noteworthy differences between men and women in terms of infection rates, disease severity, and mortality rates from COVID-19 (Cai, 2020; Muurlink, 2020). In January 2020, a preliminary analysis from 21 hospitals in Wuhan, China, discovered that 75% (126/168) of COVID-19 pneumonia patients who died were men (Xie, 2020). A study of 548 COVID-19 patients from Wuhan, China, discovered that males had a higher fatality rate (22.2%) than females (10.4%). TNF-, IL-10, lactose dehydrogenase, hsCRP, and ferritin levels were all greater in male patients, whereas lymphocyte counts were lower than in females (Qin, 2020). According to a study conducted in China between December 2019 and February 2020, men made up around 60% of COVID-19 infected individuals. As of February 11, the Chinese CDC had reported 44,600 COVID-19 cases, and the fatality rate for men with COVID-19 was 65% higher than for women. According to a survey on Wuhan children, boys made approximately 61% of children and adolescents with COVID-19 (Manoj et al., 2020). There were 13,882 cases of COVID-19 in Italy between February 21 and March 12, resulting in 803 deaths, with men accounting for 58% of all cases and 72% of all deaths. Males were 75% more likely than females to die among hospitalized COVID-19 patients. Another study, based on 3,200 COVID-19-related deaths in Italy, discovered that males died at a higher rate (70.5%) than females across all age categories. Men made up eight of the nine patients who died under the age of 40. Males had double the number of fatalities as females among COVID-19 patients aged >65 years, according to the research of COVID-19-related mortality in five European countries (Paterlini, 2020; Felix-Cardoso, 2020) (Table 3.2).

While preliminary evidence suggests that COVID-19 pneumonia affects men more frequently and severely, more research is needed to validate this. The unequal influence of male and female sex hormones on the immune system appears to be the most scientifically promising explanation for why this disparity exists (the biological hypothesis). Researchers observed differences in biological and behavioural aspects between males and females, which could explain why COVID-19 severity varied across the sexes. This difference is exacerbated by the fact that males have a higher rate of acquired comorbidities than females. COVID-19 should focus the control of

Disparity

Table 3.2 Percentage of death reported in males due to COVID-19 in major countries (Mid 2020)

Countries	Sex segregated	Deaths where sex segregated data is available	Death (% male)
USA	Yes	71,116	54
Spain	Yes	20,518	57
Italy	Yes	33,736	59
France	Partial	19,236	59
Germany	Yes	9,019	55
Brazil	Partial	54,276	59
China	Yes	2,114	64
India	Partial	3,711	64

Source Bauer et al. (2021), Wordometer (2021)

co-morbid conditions, as well as medical and social practices, in order to improve outcomes.

The living arrangements of women make them more vulnerable to the COVID-19 infection. Gender norms that define who do what appear to influence not only women's burdens but also government policy responses—they appear to be blind to women's challenges or, at the very least, try to prolong women's status as secondary earners. While gender norms and structural obstacles exhibited in economics, politics, and policy affect women's financial performance, knowing these norms, particularly structural limits, may help women mitigate their negative influence. Women may be unemployed or have no source of income, relying on male household members to meet their financial obligations. All of these risk factors for female poverty may be the result of current gender stereotypes that keep women from reaching financial independence in the first place (Rahmadhani et al., 2021).

Gender inequities played a significant role in perpetuating vulnerabilities before, during, and, most likely, after the crisis (Moser, 1993). In India, Pakistan, Nepal, Afghanistan, and Bangladesh, women hold the bulk of agricultural jobs. Poverty, according to the International Labour Organization (ILO, 2020c), is the cause of rising female agricultural work. It shows a larger gender difference in employment, more working poverty, and worse productivity, with the majority of women performing unpaid labour. In response to pandemics, however, only a few countries have established legislation concerning honorary care work (China, India, South Korea and Indonesia). In fact, South Korea is nearly the only Asian country to have implemented explicit child-care legislation. Due to a lack of temporary care givers, the Korean government has established a number of cash-based programmes to compensate for the transition of children from daycare to residential care and care for disabled family members. China, India, and Indonesia have all offered a variety of care services for elders and those with disabilities, ranging from in-home care to medical assistance and food supplements. While family subsidies helped families with finances, there appears to be a lack of direct support or process in terms of time spent by men and women sharing parental responsibilities (Rahmadhani et al., 2021).

It is likely that social safety nets were poor or non-existent in many of the nations where the pandemic had a considerable impact on women's financial well-being, to begin with, exacerbating the adverse effects of the pandemic. Gender norms that restrict women from receiving an adequate education, pursuing a good career, or being considered as secondary economic sources for their families may have contributed to their current financial difficulties (Rahmadhani et al., 2021). Because manufacturing industries such as textiles, footwear, apparel, telecommunications products, and transportation equipment, among others, have experienced the most severe trade disruptions in China, more women (34%) than men (30%) are employed in trade-disrupted manufacturing industries, hence, women are at a higher risk of losing their jobs or having their hours decreased (WTO, 2020).

Women workers in Myanmar and Bangladesh experienced similar challenges in the readymade garments industry, which employs the majority of the workforce in both countries: 65% in Bangladesh and 90% in Myanmar. Many women work as temporary employees in retail, service, and domestic industries vulnerable to consumer spending downturns such as the current crisis. In South Korea, women hold 45% of all temporary occupations, while males possess 29.4%. Because individuals eligible for paid vacation are overwhelmingly male full-time regular employees in major corporations, the predicted long-term imbalance is equally gendered (Rahmadhani et al., 2021). Women make up 44% of all informal workers in Thailand (UN, 2020). In Bangladesh, 91.8% of women work in the informal economy, including traders, shop assistants, massage therapists, domestic workers, and caretakers (UN Women, 2020). They have experienced income losses, unemployment, and restrictions on their eligibility for government-sponsored social security and stimulus programmes. Women working in small-scale agriculture are common in Afghanistan, Pakistan, and Nepal. Since the travel bans and lockdown have had an impact on the entire food chain, most notably on food production and transportation, in the coming months, agricultural producers' failure to ship their products on schedule is expected to result in a financial loss (CARE & NRI, 2020) implying that women engaged in agricultural work are likely to hit harder.

Education

COVID-19 has revealed a number of pre-existing tendencies. We have been exposed to a great deal of defects and weaknesses, such as rising inequality, the dangers of education commercialization, and the incapacity to adjust to a significant shift toward online and distance learning. On the other side, a number of positive aspects of our cultures have emerged in recent years. We see cooperation and a robust response to adversity in many communities. Many teachers, families, and children are collaborating to create extraordinary learning experiences, and their imagination, passion, and invention are amazing. COVID-19 has jeopardized public education, potentially causing division and disintegration as schools lose instructors and students who may not return when schools reopen. Furthermore, there is a degree of privatization when learning moves from classrooms to the home. Claims that the current problems and ad hoc remedies will result in long-term improvements should be viewed with skepticism.

Schools are important places for children and their families to learn about hygiene, proper handwashing, and how to deal with disturbances in their regular routines. This responsibility falls to parents, parental figures, and caregivers in the absence of access to schooling. When schools are closed, the government must step in to provide accurate and plain health information through suitable media. Nonetheless, we must acknowledge that many families and communities have come to value the teachers' efforts and competence during the trying time. The general public is becoming more aware of the multiple roles that schools play in ensuring children and teenagers' well-being, health and nutrition, and intellectual development. This improved appreciation and understanding may pave the way for a new public education system (UNESCO, 2020). Many countries have closed schools in reaction to the COVID-19 pandemic, hurting the education and learning of hundreds of millions of children. During times of difficulty, schools give children a sense of normalcy and consistency, ensuring that they have a routine and are mentally equipped to deal with this volatile situation.

UNESCO recommends that states "implement a spectrum of high-tech, low-tech, and no-tech alternatives to ensure learning continuity" to ensure that educational institutions adapt accordingly. Many teachers throughout the world are supplementing classroom instruction using online education platforms for homework, classroom activities, and research. Many youngsters benefit from using technology at home. However, not every country, neighbourhood, family, or social group has a consistent internet connection, and many youngsters live in areas where the government routinely disables the internet (Human Rights Watch, 2020). TV and radio use during COVID-19 school closures demonstrates the importance of traditional medium for education, culture, and basic information, especially for pupils who lack access to digital resources or clever gadgets. Furthermore, the COVID-19 situation highlights the critical importance of digital connections and platforms. We must regard access to information as a fundamental right in and of itself. It was closely tied to the right to health even a decade ago.

Aside from the essential variety of educational institutions, we see a tendency toward flexible learning approaches as a continuum in which schooling is conducted. From early childhood to maturity, extra formal educational facilities work more closely with a variety of non-formalized educational options. We should think about how education might be expanded to include fluidity, capillarity, and the changing circumstances of modern society (UNESCO, 2020).

Discrimination

Xenophobia and racism are on the rise around the world. Discrimination undermines the core democratic ideal of equality of rights. The attempts to highlight the link between COVID-related prejudice and increased anxiety and depression is especially relevant during the current pandemic. It exacerbates mental health distress caused by disease spread, social constraints, and financial burden. Minority rights are under attack all around the world. As the Virus spread supposedly from China, xenophobic and racist views toward Asian heritage and appearance were standard in other countries. Many people have been shunned because they are suspected of spreading the pandemic (Yenel, 2020). Sexual minorities have been subjected to rising abuse in a number of countries. Gender-based violence has skyrocketed as a result of lockdowns, depriving women of their fundamental human right to work in a safe environment.

In France, Singapore, Canada, Cyprus, Argentina, Spain, Germany, the United Kingdom, and the United States, the number of active cases, emergency calls, and nursing homes has climbed considerably. This is obviously because of a lack of basic facilities and infrastructure; digital learning has disproportionately impacted the most vulnerable and disadvantaged people, who have been excluded from national and global attempts to continue education, getting due services during the crisis.

The outbreak exacerbated the condition of individuals by limiting their access to medical care, education, political engagement, the digital environment, and the labour market (Youngs & Panchulidze, 2020). Because of the epidemic, there has been a substantial shift away from traditional educational and training environments that rely on the physical connection. Because of congestion and a general lack of resources, particularly digital devices and connectivity, the current health crisis will disproportionately affect groups that are already vulnerable in terms of knowledge and overall well-being (UNESCO, 2020).

Persons who are COVID-19 positive have regularly faced discrimination and stigma during public health crises. Since the coronavirus outbreak, numerous reports about intolerance, xenophobia, racism, and prejudice towards persons of particular descents. For example, in the United States, South Africa, Kenya, and the Philippines, people living with the Virus have faced stigma and discrimination. This has hampered their capacity to seek medical care, find work, and continue their education. Physical attacks, violent bullying in schools, vehement threats, dismissal from school or employment, and the use of derogatory language in news stories and on social media are just a few instances.

The early increase in the percentage of people experiencing COVID-related prejudice was due, in part, to discriminatory reactions to the increased number of people wearing masks or face coverings during the early stages of the epidemic. As we talked to many people travelling under some restrictions, we have known gut wrenching stories of discrimination about how the immigration officials and airport authority treat them depending on their colour and countries of origin. Asian Americans were the first racial/ethnic group to face significant discrimination, followed by African

Disparity 85

Americans in the USA. Their immigration status and mask-wearing partly explained the higher level of discrimination faced by Asians. African Americans were more likely than other non-Asian groups to face prejudice.

Wearing a mask was a consistent risk factor for discriminating linked with COVID-19, while it changed slowly over time. Frontline employees who did not wear masks, those who worked partially or entirely from home, and those who did not work were less discriminated against. People wearing masks were more likely to face discrimination prior to widespread stay-at-home orders and when mask-wearing was uncommon. Only frontline workers who wore masks were sometimes more likely to face discrimination. Researchers discovered that in the early weeks of the pandemic, people who were heavy social media users were more likely to report discrimination. They also discovered that discrimination experiences were associated with greater anxiety and depression, which is consistent with previous research linking general discrimination to poorer mental health, particularly among racial/ethnic minorities (Ullah & Huque, 2014; University of Southern California, 2020).

COVID-19 stigma could impede disease control efforts, harm mental health outcomes, and exacerbate inequities. Discrimination against people who have social or behavioural features with COVID-19 patients but may not be infected with the novel Virus was first observed online during the heightened anti-Chinese discourse. During the early phases of the epidemic, social media analyses revealed a nearly tenfold rise in the use of abusive language, and reports of in-person racist crimes against Asians increased (University of Southern California, 2020). In mid-March 2019, President Donald Trump referred to a "China virus" or "Chinese virus" and coincided with an uptick in online and in-person crimes such as robbery and harassment of Asian Americans. This virus-associated stigma toward people has been documented in prior epidemics of new viruses, regardless of illness status. Mexicans and other Latinos, for example, were avoided during the 2009 H1N1 pandemic because the Virus was linked to hog farms where migrants worked (University of Southern California, 2020).

Since the pandemic, there have been numerous allegations of racist violence against people of Asian heritage in the United States, the United Kingdom, Italy, and Spain, among others, in response to COVID-19. Mr. president Trump, inflamed anti-Chinese sentiment by the incident of naming the Virus as a Chinese Virus. Anti-immigrant politicians elsewhere in the world like as Hungary's Victor Orban and Italy's Matteo Salvini have used the pandemic to promote xenophobia (Human Rights Watch, 2020).

Population density and poverty both raise the risk of coronavirus death. For example, between January and April 2020, the UK's poorest areas in Wales had roughly 45 COVID-19 fatalities per 100,000 people, while less deprived areas had approximately 23 COVID-19 fatalities per 100,000 people (BBC, 2021). In France, death rates in the poorest quartile of the national income distribution are twice as high as in the upper quartiles (BBC, 2021). Differences in housing circumstances and occupational exposure between municipalities may explain this heterogeneity. Poorer counties in the United States have a higher death rate (60 COVID-19 deaths per 100,000 persons) than wealthier counties (48 COVID-19 demises per 1,000,000)

(Finch & Hernandez Finch, 2020). The new COVID-19 fall was significantly more extreme in the top income quintile of per capita GDP between August 2021 and October than in the other quintiles. Healthcare competence prior to the start of medical illnesses (e.g., hypertension, obesity, and diabetes) also influences death rates, all of which are connected with educational attainment (OECD, 2020a). As a result, impoverished areas bear the brunt of the attack.

Amidst enormous public health and population safety threats, states have taken exceptional measures to contain the disease—even going so far as to explicitly violate their promises. To adjust to a new environment, people's lifestyles must have dramatically transformed. All of these things were inconceivable at the beginning of 2020, but now they are commonplace. In highly populated areas, COVID-19 was linked to an increase in mortality. Having to live in a congested place is not the fault of the residents. On the other hand, residents of highly populated places were also subjected to racial discrimination.

Citizen Trust

Trust is essential in political life for politicians, law enforcement agencies, and the news media. High-profile examples of political leaders ignoring their stay-at-home orders or publicly disagreeing with or criticizing health experts can cause significant consternation and weaken public faith (Bonotti & Zech, 2021). In reaction to COVID-19, governments around the world have exerted unprecedented levels of control. While approval and trust are growing in many countries, the current enormous trust deficit is unlikely to be sustained. Hence public health experts advise that the governments must preserve confidence in order to recover from the epidemic's initial waves and build future resilience (Burrow, 2020). The politicization of topics like mandated mask wear shows how a lack of consensus may harm public health efforts and cast doubt on politicians, and law enforcement personnel tasked with enforcing compliance. In other instances, lawbreakers have been furious in their reaction towards cops executing the new legislation (Koob & Topsfield, 2020). Members of an extremist militia were imprisoned in a very rare case for allegedly attempting to kidnap Michigan's governor and put her on trial for pandemic-related brutality (Allam, 2020). Furthermore, by using framing tactics, the media can amplify the influence of public trust (or lack thereof) by prioritizing specific topics while delivering information to the wider public (Hertsgaard, 2020; Muller, 2020). A political trust may be further damaged if politicians use social media to propagate falsehoods about COVID-19 and other regulations (Kelly, 2020).

Disinformation is predicted to cost the world economy $78 billion each year, not considering societal costs (Shannon & Burrowes, 2021). It undermines public trust in government leadership and has a considerable impact on election outcomes in a number of countries. The lack of clearly defined organizations, duties, and real solutions to residents' pressing concerns and requirements exacerbates the lack of confidence.

In a number of nations, government responses to the pandemic are predicted to exacerbate corruption and graft. When confronted with critical medical requirements and limited resources, smuggling, bribery, predatory pricing, and deception are possibilities. Corruption lowers the effectiveness of healthcare treatments, particularly when large amounts of money are diverted away from high-value sectors or when patients are denied care because they refuse to pay bribes. Domestic agents and partner countries engaging in healthcare response should be aware of these hazards and resist the temptation to "do whatever it takes" in an emergency. Public unhappiness with governments may rise in the medium term as a result of the perception and reality of rising corruption. On the other hand, the crisis may force additional anti-corruption measures to be implemented. If the government's crisis management strategies elicit widespread public criticism, health governance and democratic accountability gains may be accelerated. More immediately, the prospect of widespread corruption may compel governments, democratic institutions, and international actors to take precautionary steps, particularly in countries where the epidemic has not yet struck. For example, policymakers in the United States received calls for increased monitoring as part of the country's new stimulus package. As Nigeria prepares for combatting the coronavirus, civil society groups are putting pressure on the government to implement anti-corruption measures. Additional steps include boosting the implementation of past recommendations made by advocacy organizations or raising diplomatic pressure for enhanced oversight of aid flows (Brown, 2020). Citizens want governments to take bold steps in times of crisis, particularly those that corporations frequently take. Throughout the epidemic, expectations for government performance and availability may cause institutional confidence to fluctuate.

Legislators have become increasingly responsive to the interests of economic elites in recent decades as inequality has grown (Elkjær & Klitgaard, 2021). According to Giommoni and Loumeau (2020), during the darkest days of the epidemic, voters gathered around their incumbent leaders, which may have increased political stability and loyalty to political institutions. This legitimizes the implementation of such restrictions, which may have major ramifications for political sustainability in the aftermath of the event. Lockdown tactics have been used on millions of people all around the world.

However, the extent to which these constraints affect government acceptability depends on a number of local factors, including the success of crisis management and the specific rules enacted (Elenel, 2020). Every global crisis has the potential to produce great leaders who are truthful and bold in presenting the truth. At a time when social media deception has pushed specialists to the outskirts, this is exactly what the world needs. As a result of the pandemic's unsettling reality, there is now a growing convergence in national preventative actions.

Politics of Anti-masks and Anti-vaccines

The Virus has the potential to undermine global electoral processes. Several presidential primaries in the United States have already been postponed at the state level, and candidates are campaigning in a retail-style with limited rallies (Brown et al., 2020). Furthermore, the Virus has had an impact on political participation. Protest in politics, in particular, has been a source of disagreement. Citizens in several countries have challenged government anti-virus measures such as lockdowns and mandatory stay-at-home requirements (Connolly, 2020). The internet has had an impact on political activity. On the one side, citizens in several nations have turned to the streets to oppose government initiatives to limit the epidemic, including lockdowns and obligatory stay-at-home orders (Bonotti & Zech, 2020).

The majority of republics have maintained crisis measures generally within legal limits, and their legislatures have been broad. Nations that have already experienced democratic persecution are more vulnerable to future repression as a result of COVID-19. In 61 countries, 106 elections have been postponed (IDEAS, 2021). Changes to the election schedule and voting procedures were frequently a required and acceptable component of the COVID-19 reaction, and they were implemented after the constitution was approved and validated. Election outcomes, on the other hand, are typically politicized and contested. Following the Virus's spread, certain elections saw low turnout, and a number of primaries were severely impacted. In many circumstances, leaders run the risk of jeopardizing their hold on power by postponing elections indefinitely. Ethiopia is only one example of a situation in which an adjournment could have been appropriate. While no date for the postponed election has been determined, there still remains uncertainty (Imhoff & Bruder, 2014; Youngs & Panchulidze, 2020). Of course, according to the Times of India, the Covid tsunami in India was caused by the election campaign rallies.

Political engagement has repercussions for electoral politics as well. National and regional political leaders in several countries, for example, have decided to postpone elections or rethink electoral systems. Governments took initiatives to provide social separation, healthcare, and protection during the voting process, such as expanding postal voting and implementing measures to foster social separation, wellness, and protection during the election process. Traditional customs and practices, such as handshaking, have been banned, which has an impact on advertising. Political gatherings also offer a considerable health risk for virus transmission. This became obvious after former US President Donald Trump began large-scale political campaign rallies after being hospitalized for COVID-19 therapy (Bonotti & Zech, 2020). Other politicians used virtual gatherings and events to commemorate key campaign milestones, such as the Democratic Party's announcement of their presidential nominee for the 2020 election cycle (Sprunt, 2020). COVID-19 has also influenced the content of political campaigns and elections. The significance of public health and socioeconomic and racial imbalances has grown (Ball, 2020a, 2020b), and competing parties have typically agreed on similar positions on fiscal management and government spending (McCutcheon, 2020).

Several European countries have postponed national or local elections, including Italy, the United Kingdom, Spain, North Macedonia, and Serbia. Ethiopia has also taken this move. Elections will be held in the Dominican Republic, Burundi, the Ivory Coast, Mongolia, and Malawi in the coming months, among others. The vast majority of these elections might be rescheduled. Delaying elections denies voters the opportunity to select their frontrunners (at least temporarily) at a time when leadership selection is critical. Even if elections are held, the negative impact on voter turnout, especially among the old and vulnerable, might be massive (Brown et al., 2020).

Many politicians have used COVID-19 as a reason to undermine parliamentary oversight and increase pressure on political opponents. While the public attention is focused on the health crisis, authoritarian leaders have escalated their attacks on opposition forces. The Chinese onslaught on Hong Kong democracy advocates is the most apparent form at the time, but it is far from the only cause for concern (Ullah & Azizuddin, 2020). Many countries have imprisoned opposition party leaders, activists, journalists, and healthcare professionals who have spoken out against the state's response to the coronavirus. After making critical statements about the country's crisis response, some frontline doctors in Russia mysteriously fell from hospital windows. Political opponents have been subjected to intense pressure and arrest in Thailand, Cambodia, Venezuela, and Bangladesh. Bolivian authorities used the epidemic as an excuse to threaten political opponents with prison sentences of up to ten years. Governments in the Balkans have repressed political opponents, including media outlets. In Iraq, Algeria, and Lebanon, governments have arrested 24 democratic activists for reasons unrelated to their health. In addition to addressing the health issue, Turkish authorities have increased the suppression of political and civil unrest. Kazakhstan's anti-peaceful assembly laws are egregious violations of international humanitarian law (Youngs & Panchulidze, 2020).

Globally, overall state repression has worsened in 2020 and 2021. Protests were first suppressed by curfews and movement restrictions imposed by governments. Many governments used the pandemic as an excuse. This resurgence began with frontal protests against the government's (mis)management of the pandemic and demonstrators' immediate needs, such as increased access to personal protective equipment (PPE) or financial help during the subsequent economic crisis. Protests quickly morphed into pre-crisis social movements, with pre-existing issues compounded by the pandemic's economic repercussions and government (mis)management.

As a worldwide calamity, the pandemic presented unprecedented opportunities— and reason—for those in power to impose a wide range of new restrictions and legislation. Certain individuals took the chance to strengthen their positions and consolidate power, thereby contributing to the democratic reversal. Others selectively enacted legislation or placed restrictions in order to quell resistance and minimize any challenge to authority.

In some countries, the pandemic's ramifications indirectly heightened rivalry among armed organizations, while in others, already antagonistic armed groups banded together to oppose the government's response to the outbreak. In certain cases, the coronavirus wreaked havoc on the political landscape, escalating long-standing disputes. The pandemic has direct and indirect implications on conflict dynamics. Many people thought that the crisis would lead to ceasefires in a number of the conflicts, but these hopes were mainly dashed. While the aggregate number of conflicts declined in 2019, political violence grew in more countries than it decreased, and the bulk of wars persisted. Rather, the coronavirus affected the conflict actors' incentive structures, opportunities, and timescales. In several cases, violence erupted as organizations took the opportunity to expand their operations, especially when the health crisis preoccupied state troops. In other cases, non-state players seeking greater legitimacy tried to buy local support by delivering "better pandemic governance" than their official counterparts.

The far right's anti-vaccine opportunism is disseminating an entirely new sort of global idiocy via social media, as well as in a rain of spit and insults on the street. However, it is not yet known how long it will take for COVID-19 and all its derivatives to burn out. The far-right's ignorance is considerably more resistant to science, reason, and common sense than its predecessors (Feffer, 2021).

The present anti-vax movement, which far-right political parties and organizations have hijacked, must be separated from genuine vaccine concerns. People's aversion to vaccines has been linked to a number of different qualities, such as collective trauma, scientific skepticism, and political opinions (Chen, 2021). Anti-vaccine misinformation and targeted attacks on scientists have slowed the rollout of the vaccine in many countries. The authorities seem to try to handle these issues. Anti-vaccine and anti-mask extremists have rallied around the world but mostly in developed nations. Many politicians wanted to gain some political mileage by supporting this anti-vaccine and anti-maskers propagation. The public health sector though predicted considerable vaccination resistance as the development of COVID-19 vaccines progressed. Anti-vaccine propagation has gone to that level that the WHO declared that the anti-vaccine movement is one of the world's top ten health threats (Hotez, 2021). Because anti-vax campaigns threaten to undo the progress made in the fight against vaccine-preventable diseases, despite this, the WHO notes that the reasons for non-vaccination are multifaceted and include a lack of trust, complacency, and concerns about availability to vaccinations. Between 2.3 and 3.4 million fatalities are already prevented each year, and an additional 1.5 million may be prevented if the global vaccination rate were to be improved (Hotez, 2019).

In Canada, for example, nearly three-quarters of Canadians have now been immunized against COVID-19, and the country's response to the Virus is still a heated topic of conversation among voters. Maybe that is why the most recent public health attempts to raise vaccination rates have focused on making vaccines more widely available and developing outreach programmes. This worrying convergence between the anti-vaccine movement and far-right political extremism can be seen in recent anti-vax demonstrations that have targeted schools and hospitals in particular (Gagneur, 2020).

Vaccines against the COVID-19 virus are under attack worldwide (Poggi, 2021). Getting the COVID-19 vaccine past the public's skepticism and antagonism should be a top priority. The misconception that vaccination is a violation of libertarian values must be dispelled. "Forcing vaccination is a violation of their liberal rights" is untrue, as not vaccinating puts everyone in danger. Those who oppose vaccination have no right to put others at risk. Many scientists like Poggi (2021) show how vaccination effectively promotes positive freedom using a liberal stance that weighs positive freedom against negative freedom. Some anti-vaxxers who reject the COVID-19 may be considered self-centred because of their quest for total freedom. According to defenders of negative freedom, all prohibitions and limitations on any kind of free expression should be abolished, which poses a significant challenge in public health settings (Poggi, 2021). There is a political point that the far right has hijacked the car and is driving it into oncoming traffic in support of the anti-vaccine movement. There have long been a number of detrimental views held by the far-right, both locally and globally, such as the superiority of white people, the denial of climate change, due to the rise of right-wing propagandists like Donald Trump, Jair Bolsonaro, Viktor Orbán, and Narendra Modi (Feffer, 2021).

Because of the monopoly on the vaccination industry, the wealthiest countries have been incredibly slow to give vaccines to developing nations. In Africa, for example, less than 2% of the population has been vaccinated against the most common diseases. The WHO anticipates that it will take until May 2022 for Africa to achieve 40% coverage, and until August 2024 for it to achieve 70% (WHO, 2021). This vaccine was produced quickly but has not been licensed that fast by the Food and Drug Administration and has some potentially dangerous side effects in a limited number of patients, which brings all to a concern: widespread resistance to the innovation (Feffer, 2021).

During the COVID-19 outbreak, masks have been a major point of contention. Anti-maskers' argument is that it is an infringement of their liberties and that they are ineffectual. A small but vociferous minority of the community has refused to accept the overwhelming evidence that masks help reduce the spread of coronavirus infection. Wearing a mask does not damage those who believe it does not and those who do not are enraged by those who believe it does (Stewart, 2020).

According to Stewart (2020), some people find masks irritating or suspicious that they actually work, while others have gone down a rabbit hole of conspiracy theories, including vaccines, Big Pharma, YouTube, and Bill Gates. Of course, there is a wide range of plausible causes. There are also some encouraging examples. Stewart, for example, discovered in his research that one man claims to wear a mask to the store to show respect for others who wear masks. COVID-19 will bring political ideology to its knees if public education continues to look like it did last fall. Parents' expectations for their children's return to school have shifted over the past year, but nearly all expect it to happen. Legislators who are complicit in the problem will pay the price if anti-mask legislation prevents this.

These harsh attitudes were established in the aftermath of a COVID-19 battle that appeared to be winning. Furthermore, people who back them could help build their support for the upcoming primaries and raise their national profile. By mid-summer 2020, eight states in the USA had passed laws preventing students from wearing masks in school (Black, 2021).

For the sake of their own health and that of others, why do so many people disregard public health regulations? According to one theory, people with various moral concerns respond to proposed legislation in different ways. A poll conducted by Chan (2021) found that persons with strong inclinations for caring for others and treating everyone equally are more likely to adhere to the COVID-19 recommended practices, such as wearing face masks in public. Mask-wearing may have become politicized in America early on because of government officials' face mask rules that were inconsistent, leading to an ideological divide in people's attitudes about face mask use along political lines (Faciani, 2021; Rojas, 2021). On April 3, 2020, the Centers for Disease Control and Prevention (CDC) altered its previous pro-mask attitude, resulting in a major and ongoing increase in polarization between Democrats and Republicans regarding mask-wearing. When it comes to complying with US face mask regulations, political conservatism appears to be a significant predictor of noncompliance. Democrats were shown to be much more inclined than Republicans to believe that COVID-19 poses a greater threat and hence were more likely to participate in preventative measures such as wearing face masks (de Bruin et al., 2020; Powdthavee et al., 2021).

Anti-vaccine campaigners in the United States use colonialism and eugenics. Immunization doses are currently going underused in the United States. It has been perverted by anti-vaccine advertising into conspiracy theories, exaggerated concerns, and fury at being treated like "guinea pigs" (Hotez, 2021). A large number of Africans have fallen prey to anti-vaccination propaganda as well. In Japan's capital, a modest but noteworthy protest against mask has sparked rage towards the leader of a political party who planned the protest and those who took part in it (Ryall, 2020). There were no masks on display in a protest in front of Tokyo's Shibuya Station, and many of the attendees carried posters expressing their opposition to "social isolation." They were heard chanting that it was just a cold.

In Australia, anti-vaxxers are making fake appointments at clinics in an effort to disrupt the vaccine's rollout and potentially harm vulnerable patients. According to the Royal Australian College of General Practitioners president, anti-vaxxers will "go to any length" to thwart the rollout. It is unfortunate that patients do not attend their appointments in the anticipation that the doses will be disposed of (Cassidy, 2021).

An online study performed by intelligence firm—Morning Consult—found that 17% of US citizens do not intend to obtain COVID-19 vaccine, and another 10% are undecided, implying that more than one in four people in the United States are anti-vaxxers, and the US has appeared to be ranked ranks second in terms of vaccine resistance among high-income countries (Woodward, 2021). The anti-vaccine movement has been aggressive, threatening German doctors and their staff with violence. For hard-core anti-vaccination enthusiasts to propagate internet misinformation, France is at the forefront (BBC, 2021) because the country is one of the world's most vaccine skeptical. Also to blame are the media that prefer creating a sensationalized vaccination tale rather than reporting on a factual vaccination story (Offit, 2012). The anti-vaccination movement grew stronger as a result. Anti-vaccine accusations appear to have been accepted solely because they were presented as scientifically verifiable. Many people will always hold beliefs that are not supported by evidence. Perhaps this argument is a sign of how much science is valued in our society. What we see today is that Vaccine supporters use ad hominem attacks to attack opponents. Ad hominem attacks, on the other hand, are how they get their point across. Opponents of vaccines use anecdotes about children dying as a result of vaccinations to support their argument. Vaccine proponents appeal to parents' emotions by telling heartbreaking tales of children who have died because of a lack of vaccines in order to advance their argument (Offit, 2012).

A wide range of political, societal, and personal issues are at the root of anti-vaccine campaigns. Opponents of vaccines use three tactics to combat the anti-vaccine movement: (1) questioning vaccine safety, (2) supporting individual freedom of choice, and (3) requesting research to address their concerns (Brewer et al., 2017; Powell, 2012).

The public health sector in the countries experiencing anti-vax and anti-mask extremisms has been keeping a careful eye on an exceptionally high level of resistance among a tiny portion of the population. The Anti-vax movement, however, cannot be justified on the basis of a lack of knowledge or irrational reasoning, unlike earlier vaccine reluctance. Solution aversion theory is being used to explain the growing political dispute over vaccinations (Raus et al., 2021). Individuals with varying political ideologies, according to this paradigm, see society's events differently because they are naturally opposed to specific solutions. Vaccine passports can only be implemented if the government imposes rigorous controls, which the far-right fiercely opposes (Chen, 2021) (Fig. 3.2).

Despite suffering from severe flu-like symptoms for the past ten days, "I thought I was dying," Ted Nugent, an outspoken critic of coronavirus and conspiracy theorist who has refused to receive the vaccine, has tested positive for COVID-19. As a Trump supporter, Nugent has continuously rejected the existence of the pandemic during

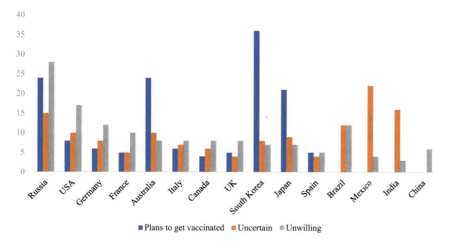

Fig. 3.2 Anti-vaccine rating (*Source* Woodward, 2021)

the preceding year. "This is not a real pandemic, and this is not a real vaccination," he stated in a Facebook video in 2020. He repeated in August a debunked conservative conspiracy idea, saying that the official COVID-19 death toll had been fraudulently inflated. They are deceiving you. Is the Centre for Disease Control and Prevention to blame (Beer, 2021)?

Conclusions

As a result of COVID-19, the world is facing unprecedented challenges, including great strain on friendships and people's connections in various aspects of their lives. Uncertainty and disruptions in social and political life will need a more nuanced understanding of how citizens should prepare for and respond to these disruptions. Under this circumstance, the political costs of the pandemic were examined in this chapter. Statesmen and other decision-makers face increased pressure to develop effective policies to control the pandemic, reduce its financial costs, and lessen its severe social and political consequences. They must achieve a balance between a wide range of opposing interests, ambitions, and goals while remaining true to sound scientific principles (Bonotti & Zech, 2021). McNamara and Newman (2020) redefine this to reflect the spirit of the world around us more effectively, emphasizing the role of identity in these shifts and shifting political control. Instead, they contend that the outbreak highlights pre-existing patterns and forces scientists to reevaluate their approach to globalization analysis.

Most importantly, we contend that globalization should be viewed as a profoundly transformative process that reorganizes identities, redefines authority and power routes, and creates new venues for contentious politics rather than a distributional war between losers and winners. It may be tempting to simply build walls and demolish globalization when countries prohibit the export of important medical commodities and governments advocate for the reshoring of global pharmaceutical supply networks. Unfortunately, the nationalist viewpoint ignores the close relationship between global economic networks and political and economic institutions. Despite this, its post-Brexit slogan remains "Global Britain," meaning that authorities recognize the UK's inability to withdraw from the world community. For Americans in need of a life-saving vaccination, international investment in a French or German company may be the greatest option. Instead of relying on current formulas, rebuilding global markets in a post-pandemic context will necessitate a reinvention of markets themselves. According to Yenel (2020), changes will occur in everyone's lives, whether permanent or temporary depending on the duration of a crisis. Transparency, solidarity, and international cooperation are critical components in overcoming adversity. It is impossible to avoid relying on science. National and global leaders must address specialists' concerns. The world has entered a new era, and the sooner it prepares for the next disaster, the sooner it will conquer it. Otherwise, the next crisis, such as COVID-19, will profoundly impact people's lives.

Human Rights Watch (2020) created a state-by-state summary of healthcare administration in regards to containing the Virus together which we argue about: (a) Initially, Chinese authorities should have taken this seriously rather taking it harshly to those people for exchanging information about outbreaks on social media, internet users were prosecuted for "rumour mongering," online discussions about the disease were outlawed, and local media coverage of the outbreak was limited. (b) In Iran, the outbreak began as a result of officials undermining public trust by forcibly suppressing huge anti-government rallies and inventing proof of the civilian airplane being shot down. As a result, Iranian officials have had to persuade the public that the government's COVID-19 pandemic actions were made in the people's best interests. The unusually high number of government employees sick with the disease and anomalies in figures given by authorities and local media sources have generated concerns that data is being deliberately underreported or is being collected and evaluated inaccurately. (c) Authorities in Thailand have reacted against global health whistleblowers and internet bloggers who have raised concerns about possible cover-ups and reported alleged wrongdoing related to surgical mask stockpiling and profiteering.

Several medical professionals have suffered legal consequences, including contract termination and license revocation, for speaking out about the country's ongoing shortage of basic supplies at hospitals. (d) Taiwan reacted rapidly to the Virus by sharing accurate information broadly. Daily news briefings and ads by health professionals have helped to reduce tensions, restore public trust, and motivate individuals to help throughout the crisis. (e) The Singapore government created and maintained thorough estimates on the number and spread of epidemics and their recovery rates on a regular basis. (f) In order to increase citizen awareness and trust, the South Korean government released health statistics, and health officials presented two daily briefings. (g) Due to internal political considerations, conflicting messages from government officials in Italy may have initially undermined the impact of public system modifications encouraging good sanitation and social isolation. The administration has held frequent press briefings to disseminate information and has launched a comprehensive public awareness campaign highlighting the necessity of protecting oneself and others against the illness.

References

Abbas, A. H. (2020). Politicizing the pandemic: A schemata analysis of COVID-19 news in two selected newspapers. *International Journal for the Semiotics of Law—Revue Internationale De Sémiotique Juridique.* https://doi.org/10.1007/s11196-020-09745-2

Abiad, A., Platitas, R., & Pagaduan, J. (2020). *The impact of COVID-19 on developing Asia: the pandemic extends into 2021* (ADB Brief No. 159). Asian Development Bank. https://www.adb.org/sites/default/files/publication/656521/impact-covid-19-developing-asia-extends-2021.pdf. Accessed 22 July 2021.

Asian Development Bank (ADB). (2020). *Asia small and medium-sized enterprise monitor 2020 – Volume II: COVID-19 impact on micro, small and medium-sized enterprises in developing asia.* ADB.

Allam, H. (2020, October 9). Michigan domestic terror plot sends shockwaves through militia world. *NPR.* https://www.npr.org/2020/10/09/922319136/michigan-domestic-terror-plot-sends-shockw aves-through-militia-world. Accessed 30 July 2021.

Alvarez, F. E., Argente, D., & Lippi, F. (2020). *A simple planning problem for covid-19 lockdown* (No. w26981). National Bureau of Economic Research.

Aratani, L. (2020, June 29). How did face masks become a political issue in America. *The Guardian.* http://www.theguardian.com/world/2020/jun/29/face-masks-us-politics-coronavirus. Accessed 30 July 2021.

Arce, J. S. S., Warren, S. S., Meriggi, N. F., Scacco, A., McMurry, N., Voors, M., ... & Mobarak, A. M. (2021). COVID-19 vaccine acceptance and hesitancy in low and middle income countries, and implications for messaging. *medRxiv, 27,* 1385–1394.

Archibold, R. C. (2010, November 17). Officials in Haiti defend focus on cholera outbreak, not its origins. *The New York Times.* www.nytimes.com/2010/11/17/world/americas/17haiti.html?scp= 9&sq=chol-era%2BHaiti&st=cse

Ball, M. (2020a, October 8). Donald Trump's COVID-19 diagnosis is forcing him to face his personal—And political—Vulnerability. *Time.* https://time.com/5897886/trump-coronavirus/. Accessed 30 July 2021.

Ball, M. (2020b, August 6). *How COVID-19 changed everything about the 2020b election.* https:// time.com/5876599/election-2020b-coronavirus/. Accessed 29 July 2021.

Baniamin, H. M., Rahman, M., & Hasan, M. T. (2020). The COVID-19 pandemic: Why are some countries coping more successfully than others? *Asia Pacific Journal of Public Administration, 42*(3), 153–169.

Bauer, P., Brugger, J., Koenig, F., & Posch, M. (2021). An international comparison of age and sex dependency of COVID-19 deaths in 2020-a descriptive analysis. *medRxiv.* https://www.medrxiv. org/content/medrxiv/early/2021/03/12/2021.03.11.21253420.full.pdf. Accessed 10 Nov 2021.

Bavel, J. V., Baicker, K., Boggio, P. S., Capraro, V., Cichocka, A., & Cikara, M., ... Willer, R. (2020). Using social and behavioural science to support COVID-19 pandemic response. *Nature Human Behaviour, 4*(5), 460–471.

BBC. (2020, June 23). Millions become millionaires during Covid pandemic. *BBC News.* https:// www.bbc.com/news/business-57575077. Accessed 12 July 2021.

BBC. (2021, October 19). Covid deaths and hospital admissions rise in Wales. *BBC News.* https:// www.bbc.com/news/uk-wales-58973788. Accessed 12 July 2021.

Beer, T. (2021). *Ted Nugent—Who called Covid-19 a scam—'Thought I was dying' from virus.* https://www.forbes.com/sites/tommybeer/2021/04/20/ted-nugent-who-called-covid-19-a-scam-says-hes-been-crippled-by-the-virus/?sh=80c2feb5534b. Accessed 10 July 2021.

Beltramo, T., Rahman, M., Sarr, I., & Nimoh, F. (2021, March 11). *Compounding misfortunes— Refugee women and girls lose even more ground during the COVID-19 pandemic.* https://www. unhcr.org/blogs/compounding-misfortunes-refugee-women-and-girls-lose-even-more-ground-during-the-covid-19-pandemic/. Accessed 10 July 2021.

Benatar, S., Sanders, D., & Gill, S. (2018). The global politics of healthcare reform. In C. McInnes, K. Lee, & J. Youde (Eds.), *Oxford handbook of global health politics* (pp. 445–468). Oxford University Press.

Bergsen, P., Billon-Galland, A., Kundnani, H., Ntousas, V., & Raines, T. (2020). *Europe after coronavirus: The EU and a new political economy.* Royal Institute of International Affairs.

Bhalla, N. (2012, July 23). Thirsty South Asia's river rifts threaten "water wars." *Reuters.* https://www.reuters.com/article/us-water-southasia-idUSBRE86M0C820120723. Accessed 1 Feb 2020.

Biswas, S. (2021). The coronavirus pandemic and global governance: The domestic diffusion of health norms in global health security crises. *Jadavpur Journal of International Relations, 25*(2), 208–234.

References

Black, D. W. (2021). *Banning masks is dangerous—For kids, in-person schooling and grandstanding politicians.* https://www.usatoday.com/story/opinion/2021/08/11/covid-19-mask-bans-threaten-kids-health-political-careers/5523964001/

Bonotti, M., & Zech, S. T. (2021). *Recovering civility during COVID-19.* Springer Nature.

Brewer, N. T., Chapman, G. B., Rothman, A. J., Leask, J., & Kempe, A. (2017). Increasing vaccination: Putting psychological science into action. *Psychological Science in the Public Interest, 18*(3), 149–207.

Brown, F. Z., Brechenmacher, S., & Carothers, T. (2020, April 6). How will the coronavirus reshape democracy and governance globally? *Carnegie Endowment for International Peace.* https://carnegieendowment.org/2020/04/06/how-will-coronavirus-reshape-democracy-and-governance-globally-pub-81470. Accessed 30 July 2021.

Burrow, S. (2020). Work: The pandemic that stopped the world. In *World economic forum.* http://www3.weforum.org/docs/WEF_Challenges_and_Opportunities_Post_COVID_19.pdf. Accessed 30 July 2021.

Cai, H. (2020). Sex difference and smoking predisposition in patients with COVID-19. *The Lancet Respiratory Medicine, 8*(4), e20. https://doi.org/10.1016/S2213-2600(20)30117-X

CARE & Nepal Research Institute (NRI). (2020). *Rapid gender analysis report on COVID 19 Nepal, 2020.* http://www.careevaluations.org/wp-content/uploads/Nepal-Final-Report_RGA.pdf. Accessed 30 July 2021.

Cassidy, C. (2021). *Anti-vaxxers trying to disrupt Australian rollout by making fake vaccine bookings.* https://www.theguardian.com/australia-news/2021/oct/05/anti-vaxxers-trying-to-disrupt-australian-rollout-by-making-fake-vaccine-bookings. Accessed 30 July 2021.

Chan, E. Y. (2021). Moral foundations underlying behavioral compliance during the COVID-19 pandemic. *Personality and Individual Differences, 171*, 110463.

Chen, S. (2021). *The anti-vax movement is being radicalized by far-right political extremism.* https://theconversation.com/the-anti-vax-movement-is-being-radicalized-by-far-right-political-extremism-166396

Clark, R. P. (2020, April 13). *When the narrative becomes the disease.* Nieman Foundation at Harvard. https://nieman.harvard.edu/stories/when-the-narrative-becomes-the-disease/. Accessed 28 July 2021.

Cohn, S. K. (2018). *Epidemics: Hate and compassion from the plague of Athens to AIDS.* Oxford University Press.

Congressional Research Service (CRS). (2021). *Global economic effects of COVID-19.* Congressional Research Service. https://fas.org/sgp/crs/row/R46270.pdf. Accessed 30 July 2021.

Connolly, K. (2020, August 3). Berlin protests against coronavirus rules divide German leaders. *The Guardian.* http://www.theguardian.com/world/2020/aug/03/berlin-protests-against-coronavirus-rules-divide-german-leaders. Accessed 30 July 2021.

Cotter, C. (2020). *From the 'Spanish Flu' to COVID-19: Lessons from the 1918 pandemic and First World War* [Blog post]. https://blogs.icrc.org/law-and-policy/2020/04/23/spanish-flu-covid-19-1918-pandemic-first-world-war/. Accessed 20 May 2020.

Crawley, H. (2021). The politics of refugee protection in a post-covid-19 world. *Social Sciences, 10*(3), 81.

Dauba-Pantanacce, P. (2020, April 20). The political implications of COVID-19. *Standard Chartered.* https://www.sc.com/en/feature/the-political-implications-of-covid-19/. Accessed 30 July 2021.

de Bruin, W. B., Saw, H. W., & Goldman, D. P. (2020). Political polarization in US residents' COVID-19 risk perceptions, policy preferences, and protective behaviors. *Journal of Risk and Uncertainty, 61*(2), 177–194.

De Vogli, R. (2011). Neoliberal globalisation and health in a time of economic crisis. *Social Theory & Health, 9*(4), 311–325.

Delanty, G. (2021). *Pandemics, politics, and society: Critical perspectives on the Covid-19 crisis.* De Gruyter. https://doi.org/10.1515/9783110713350

Denmark, A., Edel, C., & Mohandas, S. (2020). *Same as it ever was: China's pandemic opportunism on its periphery*. https://warontherocks.com/2020/04/same-as-it-ever-was-chinas-pandemic-opportunism-on-its-periphery/. Accessed 18 July 2021.

Devermont, J., & Olander, E. (2020). *COVID-19 is an African political crisis as much as a health and economic emergency*. Center for Strategic and International Studies. https://www.csis.org/analysis/covid-19-african-political-crisis-much-health-and-economic-emergency. Accessed 19 July 2021.

Ding, J., & Kananack, C. (2021). The effects of blame and politicization on responses to pandemics. *Journal of Student Research, 10*(1). https://doi.org/10.47611/jsrhs.v10i1.1320

Elkjær, M., & Klitgaard, M. (2021). Economic inequality and political responsiveness: A systematic review. *Perspectives on Politics*, 1–20. https://doi.org/10.1017/S1537592721002188

Eiran, E. (2020). *COVID-19 and great power rivalry*. http://sam.gov.tr/pdf/sam-yayinlari/The%20World%20after%20COVID19.pdf. Accessed 30 July 2021.

Equinet. (2021). *COVID-19: A magnifying glass on the vulnerabilities of women in poverty*. https://equineteurope.org/covid-19-a-magnifying-glass-on-the-vulnerabilities-of-women-in-poverty/. Accessed 9 Aug 2020.

Feffer, J. (2021, August 12). Delta variant of politics: Far right jumps on anti-vaccination bandwagon. *Business Standard*. https://www.business-standard.com/article/current-affairs/covid-19-why-is-the-far-right-jumping-on-the-anti-vaccination-bandwagon-121081200473_1.html. Accessed 6 May 2021.

Felbab-Brown, V. (2020, April 7). How COVID-19 is changing law enforcement practices by police and by criminal groups. *Brookings*. https://www.brookings.edu/blog/order-from-chaos/2020/04/07/how-covid-19-is-changing-law-enforcement-practices-by-police-and-by-criminal-groups/. Accessed 6 May 2021.

Fernandez, M., & Machado, C. (2021). *COVID-19's political challenges in Latin America*. Springer.

Finch, H., & Hernandez Finch, M. (2020). The relationship between poverty and the incidence of confirmed Covid-19 cases during the first 10 weeks of the pandemic in the United States. *Frontiers in Sociology, 5*, 47. https://doi.org/10.3389/fsoc.2020.00047

Frantzman, S. J. (2021, August 24). Toxic politicization of COVID in US has global ramifications—Analysis. *The Jerusalem Post*. https://www.jpost.com/health-science/toxic-politization-of-covid-in-us-has-global-ramifications-analysis-677573. Accessed 17 May 2021.

Gagneur, A. (2020). Respiratory syncytial virus: Motivational interviewing: A powerful tool to address vaccine hesitancy. *Canada Communicable Disease Report, 46*(4), 93–97.

García-Herrero, A. (2021). Why are Latin American crises deeper than those in emerging Asia, including that of COVID-19? In B. John, P. J. Morgan, & T. Sonobe (Eds.), *COVID-19 impacts and policy options: An Asian perspective* (pp. 362–381). Asian Development Bank.

Giommoni, T., & Loumeau, G. (2020, October 19). *Lockdowns and voting behaviour during the COVID-19 pandemic*. https://voxeu.org/article/lockdowns-and-voting-behaviour-during-covid-19-pandemic. Accessed 1 Aug 2021.

Gopnik, A. (2021, February 17). Politics, protests, and pandemics. *The New Yorker*. https://www.newyorker.com/news/daily-comment/politics-protests-and-pandemics-covid-19. Accessed 2 Aug 2021.

Guillen, M. (2020). The politics of pandemic. *Strategic Policy, Strategic Survey, 120*(1), 25–78. https://doi.org/10.1080/04597230.2020.1835086

Haffajee, R. L., & Mello, M. M. (2020). Thinking globally, acting locally—The US response to COVID-19. *New England Journal of Medicine, 382*(22), e75.

Heilbronner, H. (1962). The Russian plague of 1878–79. *Slavic Review, 21*(1), 89–112. https://doi.org/10.2307/3000545

Heisbourg, F. (2020). From Wuhan to the world: How the pandemic will reshape geopolitics. *Survival, 62*(3), 7–24.

Hertsgaard, M. (2020, March 25). The media's Covid-19 coverage proves it could also spotlight the climate crisis. *The Nation*. https://www.thenation.com/article/environment/coronavirus-media-climate/. Accessed 30 July 2021.

References

Hilotin, J. (2020). *When Russian and US scientists worked together on vaccines.* https://gulfnews.com/special-reports/when-russian-and-us-scientists-worked-together-on-vaccines-1.1597530992539

Holland, A. (2021, September 21). From bad to worse in Latin America. *The Harvard Gazette.* https://news.harvard.edu/gazette/story/2021/07/how-the-pandemic-has-affected-latin-america/. Accessed 28 July 2021.

Hotez, P. (2019). *Anti-vaccine movement is one of the ten threats to global health.* https://www.sbmt.org.br/portal/anti-vaccine-movement-is-one-of-the-ten-threats-to-global-health/?locale=en-US&lang=en. Accessed 25 July 2021.

Hotez, P. (2021). COVID vaccines: Time to confront anti-vax aggression. *Nature, 592,* 661. https://doi.org/10.1038/d41586-021-01084-x

Human Rights Watch. (2020, March 19). *Human rights dimensions of COVID-19 response.* https://www.hrw.org/news/2020/03/19/human-rights-dimensions-covid-19-response#_Toc35446577. Accessed 13 July 2021.

Imhoff, R., & Bruder, M. (2014). Speaking (un-) truth to power: Conspiracy mentality as a generalised political attitude. *European Journal of Personality, 28,* 25–43.

International Labour Organization (ILO). (2020a, June 19). *Reaching women migrant workers in Malaysia amid the COVID 19 health crisis.* https://www.ilo.org/asia/media-centre/articles/WCMS_751495/lang--en/index.htm.

International Labour Organization (ILO). (2020b). COVID-19: Impact on migrant workers and country response in Thailand. *Bangkok.* https://www.ilo.org/wcmsp5/groups/public/---asia/---ro-bangkok/---sro-bangkok/documents/briefingnote/wcms_741920.pdf. Accessed 30 July 2021.

International Labour Organization (ILO). (2020c). The COVID 19 response: Getting gender equality right for a better future for women at work. *Bangkok.* https://www.ilo.org/wcmsp5/groups/public/---dgreports/---gender/documents/publication/wcms_744685.pdf. Accessed 30 July 2021.

International Labour Organization (ILO). (2020d). *COVID-19 and the world of work* (1st ed.).

International Labour Organization (ILO). (2020e). A policy framework for tackling the economic and social impact of the COVID-19 crisis. *ILO Brief.* https://www.ilo.org/wcmsp5/groups/public/@dgreports/@dcomm/documents/briefingnote/wcms_745337.pdf. Accessed 6 July 2021.

International Monetary Fund (IMF). (2021). *World economic outlook.* IMF.

Janetsky, M., & Faiola, A. (2020, July 26). Colombian guerrillas are using coronavirus curfews to expand their control: Violators have been killed. *The Washington Post.* https://www.washingtonpost.com/world/the_americas/colombia-coronavirus-farc-eln-guerrillas/2020/07/25/927d3c06-cb64-11ea-bc6a-6841b28d9093_story.html. Accessed 28 July 2021.

Jarus, O. (2021). *20 of the worst epidemics and pandemics in history.* https://www.livescience.com/worst-epidemics-and-pandemics-in-history.html

Jiang, J., Chen, E., Yan, S., Lerman, K., & Ferrara, E. (2020). Political polarization drives online conversations about COVID-19 in the United States. *Human Behavior and Emerging Technologies, 2*(3), 200–211.

Kahf, A. (2020). *The "new normal" global governance post COVID-19.* http://sam.gov.tr/pdf/sam-yayinlari/The%20World%20after%20COVID19.pdf. Accessed 30 July 2021.

Kelly, J. (2020). *Here are the big winners and losers in our new post-Covid-19 world.* https://www.forbes.com/sites/jackkelly/2020/05/18/here-are-the-big-winners-and-losers-in-our-new-post-covid-19-world/?sh=1d34484fd2c0. Accessed 20 July 2021.

Kentikelenis, A. E., Stubbs, T. H., & King, L. P. (2016). IMF conditionality and development policy space, 1985–2014. *Review of International Political Economy, 23*(4), 543–582.

Keshavjee, S., & Farmer, P. (2014). *Blind spot: How neoliberalism infiltrated global health.* University of California Press.

Koob, S. F., & Topsfield, J. (2020, August 4). Mask-dodging woman allegedly smashed female cop's head into concrete. *The Age.* https://www.theage.com.au/national/victoria/mask-dodging-woman-allegedly-smashed-female-cop-s-head-into-concrete-20200804-p55ica.html. Accessed 30 July 2021.

Korybko, A. (2021). *Why was India excluded from AUKUS?* https://frontierindia.com/why-was-india-excluded-from-aukus/

Kreager, P. (1988). New light on Graunt. *Population Studies, 42*(1), 129–140.

Kurlantzick, J. (2021a, October 7). *How COVID-19 is transforming politics in Southeast Asia.* Council on Foreign Relations. https://www.cfr.org/blog/how-covid-19-transforming-politics-sou theast-asia. Accessed 16 Sept 2021.

Kurlantzick, J. (2021b, October 6). *Is COVID-19 shaking up politics in Southeast Asia?* Council on Foreign Relations. https://www.cfr.org/article/covid-19-shaking-politics-southeast-asia. Accessed 11 Dec 2021.

Lee, G. (2020, July 21). Coronavirus: EU leaders reach recovery deal after marathon summit. *BBC News, 21.* https://www.bbc.com/news/world-europe-53481542

Leonard, M. (2020, August 12). *The Brexit parenthesis: Three ways the pandemic is changing UK politics.* European Council of Foreign Relations. https://www.ecfr.eu/publications/summary/the_brexit_parenthesis_three_ways_the_pandemic_is_changing_uk_politics. Accessed 30 July 2021.

Levy, D. L. (2020). COVID-19 and global governance. *Journal of Management Studies, 58*(2), 562–566.

Liao, X., & Tsai, W.-H. (2019). Clientelistic state corporatism: The united front model of "pairing-up" in the Xi Jinping era. *China Review, 19*(1), 31–56. https://www.jstor.org/stable/26603249

Madiwale, A., & Virk, K. (2011). Civil–military relations in natural disasters: A case study of the 2010 Pakistan floods. *International Review of the Red Cross, 93*(884), 1085–1105.

Matta, G. (2020). Science communication as a preventative tool in the COVID19 pandemic. *Humanities & Social Sciences Communications, 7*, 159. https://doi.org/10.1057/s41599-020-006 45-1

McCutcheon, P. (2020, July 25). Coronavirus is changing the political debate on Queensland's debt, as both major parties tread the same turf. *ABC News.* https://www.abc.net.au/news/2020-07-25/coronavirus-queensland-debt-analysis-election-alp-lnp/12488184. Accessed 30 July 2021.

McNamara, K. R., & Newman, A. L. (2020). The big reveal: COVID-19 and globalization's great transformations. *International Organization, 74*(S1), E59–E77.

McNeil, D. G. (2010, November 20). Cholera's second fever: An urge to blame. *The New York Times.* https://www.nytimes.com/2010/11/21/weekinreview/21mcneil.html?auth=login-email&login=email. Accessed 9 Aug 2021.

Mellish, T. I., Luzmore, N. J., & Shahbaz, A. A. (2020). Why were the UK and USA unprepared for the COVID-19 pandemic? The systemic weaknesses of neoliberalism: A comparison between the UK, USA, Germany, and South Korea. *Journal of Global Faultlines, 7*(1), 9–45.

Moser, C. (1993). *Gender planning and development: Theory practice and training.* Routledge.

Muller, D. (2020, August 11). Tensions rise on coronavirus handling as the media take control of the accountability narrative. *The Conversation.* http://theconversation.com/tensions-rise-on-cor onavirus-handling-as-the-media-take-control-of-the-accountability-narrative-144195. Accessed 30 July 2021.

Mutapi, F. (2021, October 18). COVID-19 shows why African data is key for the continent's response to pandemics. *The Conversation.* https://theconversation.com/covid-19-shows-why-afr ican-data-is-key-for-the-continents-response-to-pandemics-169197. Accessed 30 Mar 2021.

Nakamura, D. (2020, June 24). With 'kung flu,' Trump sparks backlash over racist language—And a rallying cry for sup-porters. *The Washington Post.* https://www.washingtonpost.com/politics/with-kung-flu-trump-sparks-backlash-over-racist-language--and-a-rallying-cry-for-supporters/2020/06/24/485d151e-b620-11ea-aca5-ebb63d27e1ff_story.html. Accessed 10 Mar 2021.

Ndulu, B. (2020, August 6). *The COVID-19 pandemic and its impact on sub-Saharan African economies.* Centre for International Governance Innovation. https://www.cigionline.org/articles/covid-19-pandemic-and-its-impact-sub-saharan-african-economies/. Accessed 12 Mar 2021.

Nott, D. (2020). The COVID-19 response for vulnerable people in places affected by conflict and humanitarian crises. *The Lancet, 395*(10236), 1532–1533.

References

OECD. (2020a, November 10). *The territorial impact of COVID-19: Managing the crisis across levels of government*. OECD. https://www.oecd.org/coronavirus/policy-responses/the-territorial-impact-of-covid-19-managing-the-crisis-across-levels-of-government-d3e314e1/. Accessed 9 Mar 2021.

OECD. (2020b). *Unemployment rates, OECD—Updated: November 2020*. http://www.oecd.org/sdd/labour-stats/unemployment-rates-oecd-update-november-2020.htm. Accessed 12 Oct 2021.

Olorunnipa, T. (2020, July 14). Trump cites game show host on pandemic while undercutting doctors and questioning their expertise. *The Washington Post*. https://www.washingtonpost.com/politics/trump-cites-game-show-host-on-pandemic-while-undercutting-doctors-and-questioning-their-expertise/2020/07/13/a083ea5c-c51f-11ea-8ffe-372be8d82298_story.html. Accessed 30 July 2021.

Paterlini, M. (2020). On the front lines of coronavirus: The Italian response to covid-19. *BMJ, 368*. https://doi.org/10.1136/bmj.m1065

Poudel, K., & Subedi, P. (2020). Impact of COVID-19 pandemic on socioeconomic and mental health aspects in Nepal. *International Journal of Social Psychiatry, 66*(8), 748–755.

Powdthavee, N., Riyanto, Y. E., Wong, E. C., Yeo, J. X., & Chan, Q. Y. (2021). When face masks signal social identity: Explaining the deep face-mask divide during the COVID-19 pandemic. *PloS One, 16*(6), e0253195.

Powell, K. (2012). Facing anti-vaccine movements: Myths and facts about adverse events. *International Journal of Infectious Diseases, 16*, e57–e58.

Qin, L., Li, X., Shi, J., Yu, M., Wang, K., Tao, Y., Zhou, Y., Zhou, M., Xu, S., Wu, B., Yang, Z., Zhang, C., Yue, J., Cheng, C., Liu, X., Xie, M., & Xie, M. (2020). Gendered effects on inflammation reaction and outcome of COVID-19 patients in Wuhan. *Journal of Medical Virology, 92*(11), 2684–2692.

Rahmadhani, P., Vaz, F., & Affiat, R. A. (2021). *COVID-19 crisis and women in Asia: Economic impacts and policy responses*. Friedrich-Ebert-Stiftung.

Rajan, R. (2021). Dealing with corporate distress, repair, and reallocation after the pandemic. In J. Beirne, P. J. Morgan, & T. Sonobe (Eds), *COVID-19 impacts and policy options: An Asian perspective* (pp. 385–398). Asian Development Bank.

Raus, K., Mortier, E., & Eeckloo, K. (2021). Ethical reflections on Covid-19 vaccines. *Acta Clinica Belgica*, 1–6.

Roberts, A. (2020). Pandemics and politics. *Survival, 62*(5), 7–40.

Ryall, J. (2020, August 11). Japan has anti-mask protesters too, led by a coronavirus-denying political hopeful. *South China Morning Post*. https://www.scmp.com/week-asia/health-enviroment/article/3096902/japan-has-anti-mask-protesters-too-led-coronavirus?module=perpetual_scroll&pgtype=article&campaign=3096902. Accessed 21 Feb 2021.

Sawada, Y., & Sumulong, L. R. (2021). Macroeconomic impacts of the COVID-19 pandemic in developing Asia. In J. Beirne, P. J. Morgan, & T. Sonobe T. (Eds.), *COVID-19 impacts and policy options: An Asian perspective* (pp. 11–47). Asian Development Bank.

Scott, C. (2014). The Ebola outbreak was political-just like every disease outbreak [blog post]. *The Verge*. https://www.theverge.com/2014/12/30/7466989/the-ebola-outbreak-was-political-just-like-every-disease-outbre. Accessed 20 May 2020.

Senaratne, B. (2020, December 19). *The Covid-19 pandemic and the power rivalry in South Asia*. The National Bureau of Asian Research. https://www.nbr.org/publication/the-covid-19-pandemic-and-the-power-rivalry-in-south-asia/. Accessed 13 Dec 2021.

Shannon, J., & Burrowes, K. (2021, March 8). How governments can push towards a better tomorrow. *PWC*. https://www.pwc.com/gx/en. Accessed 30 July 2021.

Spinney, L. (2020, March 7). The world changed its approach to health after the 1918 flu: Will it after the COVID-19 outbreak? *Time*. https://time.com/5797629/health-1918-flu-epidemic/. Accessed 22 July 2021.

Sprunt, B. (2020, August 12). Harris, as Biden's running mate, says case against Trump is "open and shut". *NPR*. https://www.npr.org/2020/08/12/901462712/biden-and-harris-to-introduce-their-presidential-ticket-in-delaware. Accessed 21 July 2021.

Staniland, P. (2020). Kashmir, India, and Pakistan and coronavirus. *Carnegie Endowment for International Peace.* https://carnegieendowment.org/2020/04/14/kashmir-india-and-pakistan-and-coronavirus-pub-81529. Accessed 30 July 2021.

Stewart, E. (2020, August 7). *Anti-maskers explain themselves.* https://www.vox.com/the-goods/2020/8/7/21357400/anti-mask-protest-rallies-donald-trump-covid-19. Accessed 19 Aug 2021.

Ullah, A. A. (2014). *Refugee politics in the middle East and the Africa: Human rights, safety and identity.* Palgrave Macmillan.

Ullah, A. A. (2018). Conflicts and displacements in Syria: Exploring life trajectories of separated refugee minors. *Asian Journal of Middle Eastern and Islamic Studies, 12*(2), 207–224.

Ullah, A. A., & Huque, A. S. (2014). *Asian immigrants in North America with HIV/AIDS: Stigma, vulnerabilities and human rights.* Springer.

Ullah, A. A., & Nawaz, F. (2020). Surrogacy-led migration: Reflections on the policy dilemmas. *Public Administration and Policy, 23*(2), 157–171.

Ullah, A. A., Hasan, N. H., Mohamad, S. M., & Chattoraj, D. (2021a). Privileged migrants and their sense of belonging: Insider or outsider? *Asian Journal of Social Science, 49*(3), 161–169.

Ullah, A. A., Hossain, M. A., & Huque, A. S. (2021b). Non-conventional migration: An evolving pattern in South Asia. *Journal of African and Asian Studies, 56*(3), 00219096211008468.

Ullah, A. A., Kumpoh, A. A. Z. A., & Haji-Othman, N. A. (2021c). Covid-19 vaccine and international relations: New frontiers of vaccine diplomacy. *Southeast Asia: A Multidisciplinary Journal, 21*(1), 1–14.

Ullah, A. A., Nawaz, F., & Chattoraj, D. (2021d). Locked up under lockdown: The COVID-19 pandemic and the migrant population. *Social Sciences & Humanities Open, 3*(1), 1–5. https://doi.org/10.1016/j.ssaho.2021.100126

Ullah, A. K. M. A., Haji-Othman, N. A., & Daud, M. K. (2021). COVID-19 and shifting border policies in Southeast Asia. *Southeast Asia: A Multidisciplinary Journal, 21*(2), 1–14.

UN. (2020, June 28). *Against the odds: Stories from women in Thailand during COVID-19.* https://thailand.un.org/en/51835-against-odds-stories-women-thailand-during-covid-19. Accessed 30 July 2021.

Unicef. (2021). *Racing to respond to the COVID-19 crisis in South Asia.* https://www.unicef.org/rosa/racing-respond-covid-19-crisis-south-asia. Accessed 13 Aug 2021.

United Nations High Commissioner for Refugees (UNHCR). (2017). *Migrants in vulnerable situations UNHCR's perspectives.* https://www.refworld.org/pdfid/596787174.pdf. Accessed 30 July 2021.

University of Southern California. (2020, July 7). COVID-related discrimination disproportionately impacts racial minorities, study shows: Discrimination against people perceived to have COVID-19 increased from March to April 2020. *ScienceDaily.* www.sciencedaily.com/releases/2020/07/200707113208.htm. Accessed 12 Apr 2021.

UN Women. (2020). *Migrant workers in the Asia Pacific.* https://asiapacific.unwomen.org/en/focus-areas/women-poverty-economics/migrant-workers. Accessed 30 July 2021.

UNWater. (2019). *WASH in Health Care Facilities: Global Baseline Report 2019.* https://www.unwater.org/publications/wash-in-health-care-facilities-global-baseline-report-2019/

Vela, J. H. (2020, May 28). Trade Bazooka gets backing from main political groups in EU parliament. *Politico Pro; Draft Report,* 2019/10273(COD).

Wamsley, D., & Chin-Yee, B. (2021). COVID-19, digital health technology and the politics of the unprecedented. *Big Data & Society, 8*(1), 20539517211019440.

Weiffen, B. (2020). Latin America and COVID-19: Political rights and presidential leadership to the test. *Democratic Theory, 7*(2), 61–68.

Weis, L. (1995). Identity formation and the processes of "othering": Unraveling sexual threads. *The Journal of Educational Foundations, 9*(1), 17.

Weiss, C. (2020, March 13). Jihadists discuss coronavirus, offer advice. *FDD's Long War Journal.* https://www.longwarjournal.org/archives/2020/03/jihadists-discuss-coronavirus-offer-advice.php. Accessed 1 Aug 2021.

References

Woodward, A. (2021, September 11). The US ranks second highest among high-income countries in terms of vaccine hesitancy, one chart shows. *Insider.* https://www.businessinsider.com/vaccine-hesitancy-us-compared-other-countries-chart-2021-9. Accessed 23 Nov 2021.

World Bank. (2020). *COVID-19: Remittance flows to shrink 14% by 2021.* https://www.worldbank.org/en/news/press-release/2020/10/29/covid-19-remittance-flows-to-shrink-14-by-2021. Accessed 1 June 2021.

World Bank (2021, June 8). The global economy: On track for strong but uneven growth as COVID-19 still weighs. *The World Bank.* https://www.worldbank.org/en/news/feature/2021/06/08/the-global-economy-on-track-for-strong-but-uneven-growth-as-covid-19-still-weighs. Accessed 5 Aug 2021.

World Trade Organization (WTO). (2020a). *The economic impact of COVID-19 on women in vulnerable sectors and economies* (COVID-19 Reports, no. 2020a/10). Accessed 30 July 2021.

World Trade Organization (WTO). (2020b). *Trade set to plunge as COVID-19 pandemic upends global economy.* https://www.wto.org/english/news_e/pres20_e/pr855_e.htm. Accessed 26 July 2021.

Xinhua. (2019, September 11). *U.S. federal budget deficit exceeds 1 trillion USD for first 11 months of fiscal year.* http://www.xinhuanet.com/english/2019-09/11/c_138382147.htm. Accessed 3 Aug 2021.

Yenel, S. (2020). *The effects of COVID-19 and how to prepare for the future: Challenges of global governance amid the COVID-19 pandemic.* Council on Foreign Relations: International Institutions and Global Governance Program.

Youngs, R., & Panchulidze, E. (2020). Global democracy & Covid-19: Upgrading international support. *European Endowment for Democracy.* https://www.democracyendowment.eu/en/news/1741-global-democracy-and-covid-19-upgrading-international-support.html. Accessed 19 July 2021.

Zhuang, J. (2020, June). Mind the gap in combating COVID-19. In *East Asia forum* (Vol. 18).

Chapter 4
Pandemic, Predictions and Propagation

Introduction

The preceding chapter discussed COVID-19, its potential impact on the world, and the ways in which the world is divided by political ideology (Ma et al., 2021). This raises questions about how politicians and the media contributed to the politicization and polarization of COVID-19. This form of news coverage has the potential to cause individuals to think in ways that exacerbate political divides.

This chapter examines how the COVID-19 epidemic has altered the economy and society and how the future of labour, our social lives, education, and security will be affected. Additionally, this chapter discussed how the COVID-19 outbreak has had a significant impact on our world and killed a large number of individuals worldwide. It has had an effect on the economy and education, as well as employment losses. We attempt to forecast the end of the pandemic based on research from multiple countries. The majority of people are wondering right now: When will COVID-19 end? Is it going to end when we want it to or when we observe a significant decline in daily mortality and hospitals are no longer overcrowded?

Of course, the virus remains a problem, but it also becomes a component of the solution. Each person who recovers from a minor illness acquires greater protection against future diseases than any available vaccination. This chapter discusses how COVID-19 demonstrated that significant disparities persist between people based on their income, age, ethnic origin, gender, and where they live. People continue to face a plethora of complex, interconnected problems that impair their health and well-being. These issues are a result of social, economic, political, and environmental variables that influence people's health.

For the past two months in 2020, the coronavirus pandemic has dominated the headlines of the world news, and it has continued to do so until today and will likely do so for the foreseeable future. The crisis appears to have affected the relations of reproduction of social capital for each structural level, including public as well as mental health, employment, research, resource distribution, democracy & civil rights, human place in nature, and the quality of education. While the sequence of

---

© The Author(s), under exclusive license to Springer Nature Singapore Pte Ltd. 2022 105
AKM. A. Ullah and J. Ferdous, *The Post-Pandemic World and Global Politics*,
https://doi.org/10.1007/978-981-19-1910-7_4

events unfolds at a rapid speed of the daily news cycle, the events themselves expose the structural disparities at the root of increasing human misery, for which no rational explanation can be found. That, one might say, is how history begins to turn, the old certainties, three meals upon its kitchen table, face masks, and hospital beds all gone suddenly (Panda et al., 2021; Šumonja, 2020). Public health specialists and policy-makers have long been concerned about a pandemic emerging from the infectious virus and have issued grim warnings about the probability and ramifications of such an event, and the apocalypse has arrived. It has brought to light serious national public health challenges as well as geopolitical schisms. It has prompted discourse, pitting globalism against nationalism and populist regimes against professionals, while many world leaders' priorities have gone inward (Guillen, 2020). All of this detracts from the necessity for a concerted worldwide effort to tackle the coronavirus (Dauba-Pantanacce, 2020).

Thinking ahead, both international and domestic stakeholders are concerned about the viability of democracy. Must continually watch the pandemic's wide-ranging and fast-moving political ramifications, create swift remedies to reduce possible harm, and grab any favourable prospects the crisis may bring. Due to the global economic crisis, a second, probably even more massive wave of political instability will be unleashed. Financial inequality, unemployment, indebtedness, and poverty, as well as problems with financial institution stability, will place enormous strain on governance systems of all types. Few imagined the global financial crisis that erupted in 2008 would have such long-term political ramifications.

Nonetheless, the recession brought in the creation and development of author-itarian populism, the fragmentation of the party system, and the establishment of distinct authoritarian administrations long after the economy had recovered (Brown et al., 2020). Given its influence on population members with special and frequently complex requirements, the COVID-19 problem places a huge burden on social protec-tion budgets, and as a result, aged and dependent individuals who have long-term or chronic illnesses have been drastically affected. Those affected include the poor and marginal families, uninsured households, the homeless, informal labourers, migrants, youth, students, especially children at risk, disabled individuals, solitary people, indigenous people, and children and women in danger of domestic abuse.

Social protection accounts for 14% of total national social expenditure in OECD countries (OECD, 2019), though there are variations in social protection expendi-ture amongst OECD members. For example, social protection spending accounted for 56% of subnational spending in the United Kingdom and Ireland, compared to less than 10% in ten OECD countries. In the long run, social spending will surely grow as more welfare payments are and will be added due to rising joblessness and the number of persons requesting assistance. Unemployment benefits, guaranteed minimum income, family support, subsidized housing, disaster relief, and the ageing of the population, among other issues, will place an extra burden on sub-national government social spending (OECD, 2020a).

When confronted with a new crisis of substantially greater magnitude, it is natural for individuals and governments to be lured by the urgency of short-term domestic impacts from the epidemic. However, just as the virus knows no boundary, the

Introduction

political repercussions of the virus will definitely extend across borders and reverberate long after a health emergency has passed (Brown et al., 2020). Researchers throughout the world are evaluating the COVID-19 pandemic responses to evaluate what worked, what did not, and why. The experts cited "a few misconceptions," including the notion that policymakers must take a second seat to politics in a crisis. There are "harsh realities," one of which is that having a perfect reaction strategy is less necessary than resiliency (Smith, 2021). Trade should not be restricted, as it is critical to fund non-profit vaccine and treatment research and to keep epidemic outbreaks under control. However, political goals that contravene the notion of globalization have sabotaged such endeavours in recent years. Since the international financial catastrophe, growing geopolitical disintegration—with a world becoming multipolar and opposing 'value-systems'—has eroded global institutions' ability to coordinate a response (Dauba-Pantanacce, 2020).

The pandemic's potential to destabilize governance arrangements is owed in part to it exposing the flaws of a global financial order that appeared to be the only viable option until now. It exposes and expands institutional bottlenecks at all levels, from regional to global. It generates a significant government reaction to deal with the health issue and the related budgetary ramifications (Cotula & Schwartz, 2020). In addition to sound recommendations, a variety of factors impact lawmaking. Ideological assumptions regarding the economic or public opinion consequences of specific policies, as well as a variety of other concerns, all have a significant impact. Such fears impacting actions are difficult to prevent, and they are not necessarily prohibited. It does, however, diminish the importance of forward-thinking policy ideas, which analysts feel are critical. The failure of governments to successfully plan for recognized threats such as an epidemic cannot necessarily be attributed to ignorance. The logic of both the policymaking process and the policymaking process itself is a major impediment. Rather than assessing hypothetical possibilities—creating legislative majorities for costly and far-reaching legislation—everyday politics is controlled by the interplay of diminished interest, political contests, and more pressing issues on the daily agenda.

In ten years, as with virus prevention, every administration should be convinced that it can carry out these measures without future political support. It is possible to gather the requisite majority for effective governmental action only amid perceived crises. When danger is suspected but not yet visible, adequate preparation is uncommon. The COVID-19 outbreak is no exception (Brozus, 2020). Great crises have historically served as watershed moments in the political and social order. Economic conditions shift, alliances shift, narratives shift, and public forces reposition themselves.

Furthermore, the critical role of crises and emergency narratives in shaping public policy has received much attention (Klein et al., 2008). Legislation implemented in reaction to the pandemic in nations ranging from South Africa to India, Colombia, and the United Kingdom has put existing governance principles to the test, affecting human rights, commercial operations, markets, and cross-border trade. While overcoming the acute crisis must take precedence, these issues entail a study of the fractures and continuity of the political and economic structure. In light of the pandemic's peculiar circumstances, they call for a crisis-ridden political economy (Tsoukalis, 2012). This shows how different government officials reposition themselves and renegotiate ties. As the crisis deepens and, in the long run, so will the debate and actual action, with potentially far-reaching ramifications across a range of policy domains.

According to all global analyses, it appears that COVID-19 sparked an economic downturn comparable to that which followed World War II. Even if an effective vaccine is available at the right time, it is unlikely to lead to a quick recovery from COVID-19's global economic havoc. Because of this, economic arguments have switched more and more to measures for encouraging this recovery. Few studies have suggested the trade-offs associated with various policy options at the global level (Fernando & McKibbin, 2021). A study by McKibbin and Vines (2020) looked at the role of international collaboration in fostering economic recovery and the manner in which it can improve global economic outcomes.

The Economic Landscape

The COVID-19 epidemic has been connected to a significant increase in unemployment in a number of countries (Ullah, Hossain, & Huque, 2021). People around the world have lost jobs or had their working hours reduced as a result of COVID-19, which has been plaguing the global economy for the past years. According to the most current ILO Monitor, 114 million jobs would be lost by 2020, resulting in nearly four times the number of working hours lost during the 2009 financial crisis when combined with work-hour reductions within employment, and a total of 255 million full-time jobs will be lost in 2020, resulting in a $3.7 trillion loss in labour income (Ayittey et al., 2020; ILO, 2020c). The ILO's worst-case scenario from spring 2020 predicted a loss of between $860 billion and $3.44 trillion in labour revenue for the entire year. A total of 525 million working hours were lost in the second quarter of 2020 due to wide-ranging lockouts. Millions of individuals had returned to work in 2021 or had transitioned to working from home by the end of 2020, and global working hours have not come back in 2021 (Richter, 2021).

When it comes to deploying automation and artificial intelligence, COVID-19 has the ability to speed up the process. Historically, firms have used automation and reorganization of labour processes to decrease costs and eliminate uncertainty during economic downturns. More than two-thirds of the 800 top executives polled in a July 2020 global survey reported that they were increasing their investment in automation and artificial intelligence. By June 2020, China's robot output will be more than before the outbreak. By 2021, China is expected to account for 45% of the global exports of industrial robots, up from 39% in 2020. There are already 97 industrial robots for every 10,000 manufacturing workers in China—half the amount in the United States and one-seventh in South Korea (Fannin, 2020). China's first robot-run ward began construction on February 28 to prevent Wuhan Wuchang Hospital workers from being infected with COVID-19. After the Chinese government

The Economic Landscape 109

enforced a lockdown on Wuhan on January 24, every Chinese robot company tried to contain the virus since it first appeared on the scene. They were pitching robotic ward sanitization, temperature monitoring, and drug dispensing to hospitals in a matter of weeks done by robot (O'Meara, 2020).

According to the latest job loss figures, coronavirus's economic impact will continue to be long-lasting, and Trump's concept of rapid, V-shaped recovery is at odds with what people across the country are facing. Consider greater government investment and long-term solutions in addition to those being examined by Congress for short-term solutions (Cassella, 2020; Parker et al., 2020).

Since the coronavirus outbreak began, these additional services have been more popular among low-income Americans. Many lower-income adults have used money from their savings or retirement accounts to pay for expenses during this time period, and many more have borrowed money from friends or family (35%) and received food assistance (25%) from food banks and charitable organizations (35%), a third of the population. Middle-income people use savings or retirement accounts to pay for their expenditures; 11% borrow from family and friends; 13% get food from a food bank or charitable organization, and 7% get government food assistance. Moreover one-fifth of those in the upper-income bracket have used savings or retirement funds to pay their obligations since the coronavirus pandemic began (Parker et al., 2020).

Job losses or wage reductions due to the coronavirus are significantly more common among people who have used more resources. Only 17% of those whom the coronavirus outbreak has not touched have utilized savings or retirement funds to pay their bills, compared with 46% of those who have been laid off or have had their income decreased. Some 24% of those who have lost a job or had a fall in their income report borrowing money from family and friends; 20% report getting food from a charity; and 18% report receiving government food aid (Parker et al., 2020) (Table 4.1).

Table 4.1 Estimated job and wage income losses due to COVID-19

	Employment ($ million)	Wage income ($ billion)
World	158.1–242.1	1,201.2–1,832
Developing Asia	108.7–166.3	347.5–532.8
Central Asia	1.9–3.0	3.4–5.4
East Asia	65.1–98.8	291.3–445.7
Southeast Asia	11.6–18.4	25.0–39.0
South Asia	30.0–45.9	27.6–42.4
The Pacific	0.1–0.2	0.2–0.3
United States	9.0–13.5	402.7–611.2
Europe	16.5–25.1	272.1–415.5
Rest of the world	23.9–37.2	178.9–272.9

Source Sawada and Sumulong (2021) (with permission)

A growing number of companies are using automation and artificial intelligence (AI) to minimize labour density and respond quickly when demand increases. There is a common denominator throughout this automation use cases, and our study indicates that work environments with a high level of human connection are predicted to have the greatest acceleration in automation and AI adoption. There may be a more significant shift in the mix of work in an economy due to COVID-19-accelerated trends than projected prior to the pandemic.

Following the pandemic, we find that each of the eight economies may generate a significantly different mix of jobs. According to our pre-COVID-19 forecasts, food service, customer service, and low-skilled office support will be the hardest hit by the pandemic. As e-commerce and the delivery economy grow, warehouse and transportation jobs may flourish, but these gains are unlikely to compensate for the loss of many low-wage jobs. Customers and food services are forecast to lose 4.3 million jobs in the United States, while the transportation sector is expected to add 800,000 employment (Cox, 2021). Increased attention to health as people get older and wealthier, as well as a growing need for individuals who can design, implement, and manage new technologies, are all factors that could lead to an increase in the need for healthcare and STEM experts.

By 2020, the Asia–Pacific Employment and Social Outlook 2020: Navigating the Crisis to a Human-Centred Future of Work anticipates that economic implications from the COVID-19 outbreak will result in the loss of 81 million jobs in Asia–Pacific. Compared to 2019, employment numbers fell in practically every economy, with quarterly statistics available in 2020.

The economic crisis has had a wide-ranging impact, with millions of people being forced to work fewer or no hours as a result. In the second and third quarters of 2020, working hours in Asia and Pacific working hours are expected to fall by 15.2% and 10.7%, respectively, compared to pre-crisis levels (ILO, 2020b). As a result of fewer paid hours worked, median earnings have decreased. Employee income in the Asia–Pacific area is expected to shrink by up to 10% in the first three quarters of 2020, which is equivalent to a 3% GDP decline (ILO, 2020). As a result, there is a rise in the number of working poor. Preliminary research suggests that between 22 and 25 million people may fall into working poverty by 2020, bringing the total number of working poor in the Asia–Pacific region to between 94 and 98 million. There's a significant possibility that the cause of unemployment was exogenous (or outside the individual's control) due to the COVID-19 epidemic, which provides an unparalleled opportunity to examine the psychological effects of job loss (Posel et al., 2021).

COVID-19 pandemic-related regulations are expected to cost 4.5 million African aviation and aviation-related jobs in 2020 out of 7.7 million total aviation-related positions in Africa. Approximately 40% of Africa's 440,000 aviation jobs are anticipated to vanish by the end of 2020, and an estimated 58% drop in Africa's GDP from pre-pandemic levels can be attributed to the decline in aviation's contribution to the continent's economy (Anadolu Agency, 2020). "Millions of people would suffer social and economic effects due to the worsening of African air connectivity." As a result of a lack of money, many people are unable to receive social services. Governments must safeguard the continent's reunification to the fullest extent possible. There

The Economic Landscape

will be a loss of many jobs and an economic collapse if the borders are closed or quarantine procedures are put in place to restrict air travel (Anadolu Agency, 2020) (Table 4.2).

Job losses are going to lower global wage income by $1.2 trillion to $1.8 trillion. An estimated 109 million to 166 million jobs would be lost in emerging Asia by 2020, making up roughly 70% of all global job losses. Between $348 billion and $533 billion in wage income losses are expected in the region, accounting for about 30% of the global losses (Table 4.1). However, not all jobs are affected in the same way. It has been disproportionately impacted by low-skilled workers, women, informal sector workers, and international migrant workers (Sawada & Sumulong, 2021).

Interestingly, online sales organizations suffered more permanent or temporary employment losses than those that did not implement the technology (Sonobe et al., 2021). The researchers also revealed that companies that grow their online sales

Table 4.2 Estimated job and wage income losses due to COVID-19 (GDP)

	GDP (%)			GDP loss ($ billion)		
	Better	baseline	worse	Better	baseline	worse
2020						
World	−5.5	−7.2	−8.7	4,757	6,165	7,441
Developing Asia	−6.0	−7.8	−9.5	1,394	1,818	2,211
Central Asia	−9.3	−11.9	−14.2	34	43	51
East Asia	−4.6	−6.0	−7.4	761	999	1,223
Southeast Asia	−8.6	−10.9	−12.7	253	320	374
South Asia	−10.0	−13.2	−16.3	443	353	560
The Pacific	−7.0	−8.7	−9.6	2	3	3
United States	−4.9	−6.4	−7.8	1,038	1,349	1,634
Europe	−7.9	−10.2	−12.2	1,488	1,913	2,285
Rest of the world	−3.6	−4.6	−5.6	836	1,084	1,310
2021						
World	−3.6	−4.9	−6.3	3,108	4,234	5,407
Developing Asia	−3.6	−4.9	−6.3	855	1,148	1,470
Central Asia	−6.2	−8.6	−11.1	23	31	40
East Asia	−2.4	−3.3	−4.2	402	547	698
Southeast Asia	−6.1	−8.4	−11.0	178	246	322
South Asia	−7.0	−9.4	−11.8	240	322	406
The Pacific	−3.8	−5.6	−7.8	1	2	3
United States	−3.3	−4.5	−5.8	696	947	1,212
Europe	−5.1	−7.0	−9.0	956	1,311	1,697
Rest of the world	−2.6	−3.5	−4.4	612	828	1,027

Source Sawada and Sumulong (2021) (with permission)

have a greater chance of cutting back on their workforce and a lower chance of increasing their workforce. Initial effects on employment and business viability were profound due to the epidemic. There was a great deal of eye-opening results from their investigation.

Economic stimulus packages with considerable government investment were implemented in many Asian countries to restrict the progress of the COVID-19 virus, as well as to improve health care. Among them are the 10 ASEAN nations, Japan, the People's Republic of China, and South Korea. Within one month of the World Health Organization deeming COVID-19 a pandemic, each government developed substantial policy packages to prevent the virus' spread and maintain economic activity (on March 11, 2020) (Shinozaki & Rao, 2021). In a number of Asian countries, MSMEs and industries harmed by natural disasters were exempt from social security obligations (for example, Cambodia, Japan, Malaysia, the PRC, Thailand, and Viet Nam). Value-added tax (VAT) exemptions and reductions have also been granted in a number of countries (Indonesia, Malaysia, the PRC, Singapore, and Viet Nam). To help small business owners and self-employed individuals, they offered a wide range of tax breaks or exemptions. Tourist destinations like Bali benefited from the federal government compensating local governments for lost tax revenue caused by a 6-month suspension of tax payments (Shinozaki & Rao, 2021). After the lockdown, the Philippine economy saw a significant drop in domestic production and consumer confidence in the country's economy (Shinozaki & Rao, 2021). Predicted massive economic losses when paired with enterprise finance limitations (ADB, 2021a, 2021b) (Fig. 4.1).

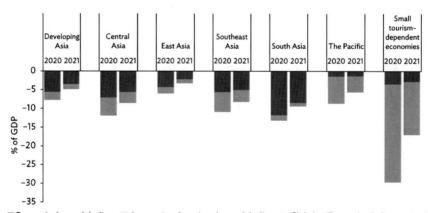

Fig. 4.1 COVID-19 estimated impact on developing Asian economies (*Source* Sawada & Sumulong, 2021 [with permission])

Politics and Electoral System

COVID-19's impact on global politics, economics, and the role of technology has sparked a lot of discussion since its breakout. However, governments and society's response to the epidemic will have an impact on these ramifications. The pandemic has been going on for about two years. There is now a clear picture of how countries and political systems have dealt with the effects of the change. Global politics may be affected and will be affected by the epidemic's impact.

The epidemic has had a profound impact on the state's global politics. Even once the pandemic is over, we may expect the Gig government to be back with a vengeance, which is unlikely to change. Implying that additional government action will be required to distribute vaccines. As shown by numerous states' economic stimulation programmes, increased state intervention is also needed for economic recovery, particularly in South Asia and Africa. The "minimal government and maximum governance" campaign pledge of Prime Minister Narendra Modi has lasted less than a year. While the larger government is inevitable, "ideal" governance is not. Despite this discrepancy, the record remains unbeaten. States and other constituent units have had a considerable impact on the central government's authority, even in federal systems, due to the spread of the pandemic. The pandemic in India gave the federal government an excuse to go above and beyond its constitutional bounds. The pandemic's crisis-like aspect quelled dissent even in states that the BJP did not rule. With the Centre's refusal to meet its obligations to compensate for GST collection losses, the states' financial dependence on the Centre has greatly increased. This has changed the power balance from the Centre to the states, significantly increasing their financial reliance on the Centre. Union government has leveraged its stronger authority to push through reforms in agriculture, education and health care, all traditionally state responsibilities, with only modest and occasional opposition. Regardless of the country's constitution, post-pandemic India is likely a more unified state (Benzian et al., 2021; Reddy, 2021). "Fissiparous tendencies," a phrase developed in our country's early years, are a result of this, and they will only get worse (Saran, 2020).

Unprecedented events are taking place at this time. An increase in worldwide awareness has been brought about by the COVID-19 pandemic and its economic repercussions. Prejudice and discrimination have lasted longer than the Berlin Wall. Everyone understands that the difficulties we all confront are systemic and that big changes are needed to address them. There is no going back to normal in the face of the pandemic's social effects, economic policies, institutionalized racism, and dangers to global sustainability (Bradford, 2020).

Leaders have two key tasks during a crisis: to deal with the current problem and to prevent a repeat of the incident. As a case in point, the COVID-19 outbreak serves as an excellent illustration. In the immediate aftermath of an outbreak, we must save lives and improve our ability to respond in the long term. Both issues have long-term ramifications, but the first is more urgent. Muhyiddin's Malaysian government is not exempt from this rule (Yaakop et al., 2020).

A substantial body of literature has proven that election participation is influenced by a range of barriers that increase the cost borne by individual voters; a phenomenon is known as the voting calculus framework, from the early works of Downs (1957) and Riker and Ordeshook (1968). The calculus of voting is often characterized as the expected benefit of voting (satisfaction with the preferred candidate multiplied by the likelihood of being the deciding voter) plus the satisfaction of voting unrelated to election outcomes minus the cost of voting (Mueller, 2003). Under this paradigm, the cost of voting has two major components. On the one hand, voters' costs in preparing to vote, such as the time and resources spent learning about candidates, their platforms, and the important election issues (Converse, 2000). On the other hand, people suffer a direct cost associated with voting, albeit a little one (Aldrich, 1993), which includes the time required to drive to the polling place, wait in line, and cast the ballot. Numerous studies have identified a variety of factors influencing electoral turnout, including transportation costs (Fauvelle-Aymar & François, 2018), election-day weather (Gomez et al., 2007), the number of simultaneous ballots, the day of the week, and the holiday period, as well as voting technology and voting processes available (Fujiwara, 2015).

In mid-July 2020, the Democratic Party nominated Joe Biden and his running partner in Milwaukee, while the Republican Party is prepared to renominate Donald Trump in Charlotte, North Carolina. Trump was leveraging the roaring economy to bolster his case for re-election at his usual rallies, while Biden's plea for a return to normalcy fails to inspire audiences (Ball, 2020a, 2020b). Trump's supporters have continued to promote conspiracy theories about the Biden family's connection in Ukraine, prompting Democrats to demand for a second House impeachment. Both parties are waging a frantic campaign across the country, knocking on millions of doors in an effort to turn out voters in November. Trump has become an unstoppable force and an inevitable fact of national politics and American life during the last four years of his tenure. Now, he's been displaced as the campaign's main character by a virus with no calendar, ideology, or political goal. The virus has caused a seismic upheaval in the most fundamental act of American democracy: how Americans choose the President charged with ending the pandemic's reign of destruction, dealing with its aftermath, and building the society that rises from its ashes. And, like with many other changes caused by the coronavirus, the practice of American politics may never be the same again (Ball, 2020a, 2020b). As a result of COVID-19, at least 79 countries and territories have agreed to postpone national and subnational elections, with at least 42 countries and territories deferring national elections and referendums. Despite doubts about COVID-19, at least 142 countries and territories have agreed to hold national or subnational elections, with at least 120 holding national or referendum. At least 57 countries and territories have held elections that were originally postponed due to COVID-19 concerns (Fig. 4.2), with at least 29 holding national elections or referendums (International Institute for Democracy and Electoral Assistance, 2021).

The epidemic could cause changes in election and voting processes, increasing resistance to future shocks. The number of early voting and vote-by-mail alternatives

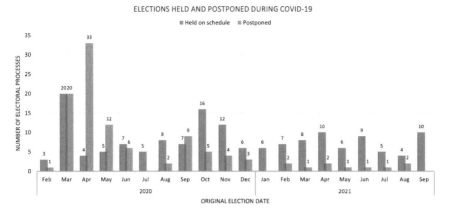

Fig. 4.2 Election held and postponed during COVID-19 (*Source* International Institute for Democracy and Electoral Assistance [IDEA], 2021 [with permission])

has been increased. Capital investments in voter education, growing reliance on online voting technologies, and voter fixation online are all plausible results.

Adopting steps such as allowing residents to vote from the comfort of their own homes or hospitals. Significant changes in election administration, on the other hand, will introduce new complexities and risks, necessitating careful planning. Electronic voting machines are subject to hacking and prefixed results, raising concerns about foreign interventions. And cross checking is not possible. Certain developments may be impossible to implement in countries with limited technological capacity. Countries that have pioneered ground breaking voting technology may be able to give insight on this topic (Corpuz, 2021; Brown et al., 2020). There has been a surge in the number of new online democratic forums. Initiatives that involve individuals in online parliamentary debates are among them. Brazil, Colombia, Albania, and the Maldives have all changed their laws to allow remote digital labour. Chile and Singapore have changed their constitutions to permit online parliamentary debate. For example, Armenia, Indonesia, Guatemala, and Kosovo have created social media platforms to boost public involvement. Numerous countries have discussed ways to increase electronic voting in public and parliamentary elections while also addressing digital threats to make these activities safer (Youngs & Panchulidze, 2020).

According to Freedom House's seminal assessment of political rights and civil freedoms, the pandemic has exacerbated the 15-year fall in democracy globally. Approximately 45% of all countries and territories that experienced an erosion of freedom in 2020 were affected by the epidemic. With the introduction of a new vaccine, this year's unequal and politicized vaccination distribution threatens to exacerbate the health catastrophe and wreak havoc on global democracy (Slipowitz, 2021). In the event of a public health emergency, restrictions on fundamental rights, such as freedom of movement and assembly, may be justified, transitory, and nondiscriminatory. COVID-19, on the other hand, was regularly exceeded by governments. In order to enforce lockdown measures, limit free speech, and implement extensive state of emergency decrees that erase due process rights and boost presidential authority, governments all over the world have turned to violence (Slipowitz, 2021).

If we think of democracies as vertical and horizontal accountability systems, we can better understand the COVID-19 problems for liberal democracies (Lindberg, 2013; Schedler, 1999). Civil freedoms and political liberties must be in place to ensure political authorities' responsibility so that citizens can live their lives in freedom and express themselves constructively (Dahl, 1971; Merkel, 2004). Liberal democracy is characterized by horizontal responsibility as well as vertical accountability, which is important for the protection of minorities' rights and the promotion of pluralistic modalities of political decision-making (Coppedge et al., 2011).

The democratic trade-off reveals itself at two distinct levels of pandemic management in contradiction to these principles. When it comes to halting the spread of the virus, measures that restrict fundamental civil liberties, which are safeguarded in liberal democracies and can only be diminished under extremely rare circumstances, are the most successful at doing this (Coppedge et al., 2011). Second, the requirement to respond swiftly is in conflict with the principles of separation of powers and the rule of law, which normally govern state activity and provide horizontal accountability (Zwitter, 2012: 100). Consequently, the administration now assumes legislative functions traditionally held by parliament.

COVID-19-related actions fall under two major categories that contravene democratic ideals. Methods to prevent the spread of the virus through physical contact between individuals that restrict individual freedom but are incompatible with fundamental civil and political rights such as freedom of movement or assembly are first examined. Travel restrictions on both local and international levels, a ban on public meetings, and rigorous "stay-at-home" laws are among these measures (Goetz & Martinsen, 2021; Nicole & Orsolya, 2021).

Second, we examine power concentration, which refers to the transfer of legislative authority from parliament to the executive in order to enhance the executive's ability to effectively implement COVID-19-related policies. During times of national hardship, the established principle of the separation of powers is challenged by the use of such means of evading regulations. Even in certain nations where democracy has been eroded, the executive power has been increased because they have gained control of their own media. So-called fake news restrictions that restrict media coverage of COVID-19 and the government's response to COVID-19 violate the fundamental right to free expression and information (Goetz & Martinsen, 2021; Nicole & Orsolya, 2021).

Freedom of Expression

At least 83 states have used the COVID-19 outbreak to justify violating citizens' rights to free expression and peaceful assembly (Human Rights Watch, 2021a, 2021b). Government authorities have assaulted, imprisoned, prosecuted, and in some cases killed opponents, dispersed peaceful protests, closed down media outlets, and enacted unclear laws criminalizing speech they believe is damaging to public health. Journalists, activists, healthcare workers, political opposition groups, and others who have questioned the government's handling of the coronavirus have been among those killed. Governments should fight COVID-19 by encouraging people to mask up rather than shut up. Beating, detaining, prosecuting, and silencing peaceful critics violates fundamental rights, including the right to free expression, and does nothing to stem the pandemic (Human Rights Watch, 2021a, 2021b).

Human Rights Watch (2021a, 2021b) urges that governments and other state authorities should immediately cease unwarranted restrictions on free expression in the name of curbing COVID-19 and hold those responsible for significant human rights breaches and abuses accountable. During its session beginning February 22, 2021, the United Nations Human Rights Council should commission a new report from the UN High Commissioner for Human Rights focusing on states' compliance with human rights obligations in response to COVID-19, including the impact of restrictions on free speech and peaceful assembly.

Human Rights Watch (2021a, 2021b) investigated responses to the COVID-19 outbreak of several governments around the world and discovered that unlawful interference with free expression was one of the most common types of overreaches. Violations were widespread in various countries. Hundreds of thousands of people were harmed as a result of government abuses in countries like China, Cuba, Egypt, India, Russia, Turkey, Venezuela, and Vietnam. Individuals are still being detained in certain countries, like Bangladesh, China, and Egypt, for criticizing the government's response to COVID-19 (Human Rights Watch, 2021a, 2021b).

Following the outbreak, democratic societies around the world must increase their coordination. Democracy and COVID-19 necessitate a truly global response spanning all continents. Countries such as Canada, New Zealand and Korea may participate in this collaboration since they have successfully responded to crises in the past, particularly by retaining a functional democratic framework during the crisis. These countries, potentially joined by one or two of Europe's and other democracies' best performers, may create the framework for an international democratic push in the coming years. A global campaign could promote Asian, African, and Latin American countries' strong governance practices and governance lessons.

A large (virtual) event could kick it off. This global coordination must prioritize democratic learning, including more effectively showcasing democracy's benefits in times of crisis, forging consensus positions when civil liberties are challenged, and, in some situations, coordinating programmatic actions on the ground. It should also engage in long-term planning: democratic leaders should share lessons learned to better prepare for crises and finish reducing their impacts. By framing a project in these terms, it will be easier to construct a narrative that proves democracy's compatibility with COVID-19 goals, dispelling the idea that political liberty and high-quality health care are mutually contradictory. One of the most puzzling challenges raised by the epidemic would necessitate even greater international cooperation: a China emboldened to express itself more assertively beyond its boundaries and whose model may be increasingly replicated by others. Even though it is a common procedure elsewhere, this will be crucial in Hong Kong (Youngs & Panchulidze, 2020).

Governments should protect freedom of expression to the greatest extent practicable while exercising control only to the extent permissible by international law. Governments should ensure that the public receives accurate, timely, and human-rights-compliant COVID-19 information. This is especially important when dealing with incorrect or misleading information.

COVID-19 materials should be offered in a range of languages and accessible to people with limited or no literacy skills. This should include good sign language comprehension for television announcements, as done in Taiwan; websites that are truly accessible to those with visual, hearing, learning, or other disabilities; and phone line services with message capacity for deaf or blind people. Written communications should be as brief as possible. Children should be given age-appropriate information to help them take precautionary measures. Health information is particularly delicate, and disseminating it online can endanger people, particularly those who are already marginalized or on the periphery of society. Legal safeguards should control rights-based; personal health data must be handled and stored correctly. It is vital to preserving unfettered and reliable internet access, as well as to take steps to ensure that people with low incomes have access to the internet. During the pandemic, additional efforts may be undertaken to relax data restrictions, enhance speeds, and abolish eligibility limits for practically all low-income targeted programmes (Human Rights Watch, 2020).

Prejudice and Sigma

Today, humanity is confronted with one of the century's most pressing issues. The novel coronavirus spread to the point of being declared a pandemic (Bhanot et al., 2021). The rise of the COVID-19 outbreak has concerned people all around the world. People are saddened by what is happening to them, as well as by the misfortune of others, particularly the disadvantaged. People's everyday routines change dramatically. Aside from worry, anxiety, and sadness, people's frustration about the future has skyrocketed. In the midst of such a rapid surge of COVID-19 (Earnshaw, 2020), one of the most severe issues that must be addressed promptly is the epidemic related stigma.

It has been shown that individuals and groups are shifting from a wish to live in mutual connectedness to a desire to stigmatize individuals, groups, and nations seen as potential sources of viral infection. In other words, the pandemic appears to be causing othering on both a global and local scale, resulting in huge social capital loss. The stigmatizing behaviours in this context are driven by the adage "better safe than sorry" (Bhanot et al., 2021), which describes how fear of the unknown and uncertain (Logie & Turan, 2020) accounts for negative attitudes toward persons who are infected or suspected of being affected, as well as those suspected of spreading the virus.

Since the outbreak of the pandemic in India, for example, there has been a negative attitude toward people infected with the virus. COVID-19 patients are accused of being misinformed and reckless, and hence, they are considered responsible for developing the virus (Earnshaw, 2020; Kalpana et al., 2021). Patients with COVID-19 were categorized as active coronavirus spreaders and treated as passive disease acquirers (Logie & Turan, 2020). Hence, society reacted badly by enacting a range of harmful measures (including posting harsh comments on social media, prohibiting them from entering residential areas, and spreading stories about them based on their religion, class, and caste). Because of the virus's peculiar character, the devaluation associated with the COVID-19 mark is irreversible (Bhanot et al., 2021). That is possibly why the virus's stigma is so severe that even those who have previously been diagnosed continue to be stigmatized (Logie & Turan, 2020), and even after overcoming the sickness, they have been unable to overcome social rejection. They claim to be treated as untouchables, subjected to humiliating insults and having fingers pointed at them and their families; their area has been dubbed "corona wali gali" (corona street), and the resulting difficulty has prompted them to sell their own home. Fear has become so ubiquitous among the public that they have turned to scapegoats, most notably the poor, labourers, daily wagers, and migrants (Bhanot et al., 2021).

COVID-19 has been generating headlines since January 1, 2020. The dynamics of worldwide migration were flipped on their heads by early March 2020. The situation is dire, with most planes grounded and travel restrictions constraining people to their homes and neighbourhoods (Ullah et al., 2021). The COVID-19 pandemic has exacerbated these imbalances. Individuals on society's periphery are increasingly cut off from the benefits and opportunities enjoyed by the majority of us. Migration-related inequalities are surfacing, though migration can help reduce inequality by redistributing resources on a national, regional, and global scale. Its equalizing effects are unknown, not least since there are significant variations in mobility, the right to be protected, and access to jobs, education, and health care (Black et al., 2005). Existing spatial, economic, and social injustices, such as gender, age, and income inequality, are typically reflected and exacerbated by rights and opportunities for population increase (Crawley, 2019). COVID-19 is known as the "great equalizer" since it may infect anyone, regardless of status or socioeconomic class (Crawley, 2020). Local governments and officials are making progress in implementing the lockdown, frequently in collaboration with community leaders. The majority of people were aware of the procedures put in place in their communities to avoid illness spread. To name a few, providing hand-washing stations, prohibiting strangers from entering communities, encouraging inhabitants to stay at home, increasing social distance, and coordinating for aid where it was most needed. According to others, despite the fact that mosque organizations were vital to the lockdown's effectiveness in the majority of places, it was difficult to persuade religious leaders to help with the lockdown. The general public is afraid of being limited by the municipal administration or by community members acting alone (BIGD, 2020).

COVID-19-related prejudice and stigma must be addressed early as a vital component of global pandemic response efforts. During the response, people from vulnerable groups, such as ethnic and racial minorities, must be safeguarded and stigmatized as little as possible. Data from various sources suggest that COVID-19 is putting these people at risk of significant morbidity and mortality. All community sectors must be included and contribute to the creation of COVID-19 context-specific community health solutions. Countries can draw on three decades of experience working with HIV-positive people's networks, vulnerable populations, and women's groups to guide and support community-based community health responses to COVID-19 (UNAIDS, 2020). Governments must act quickly to protect families and organizations suspected of being implicated in COVID-19, conduct full investigations into all incidents, and prosecute perpetrators. Governments must ensure that COVID-19 measures do not discriminate against or target specific ethnic or racial groups and that marginalized groups, such as people with disabilities or special needs, are included and treated with dignity. Governments must ensure that people with disabilities or special needs have equal access to emergency services as the rest of the community. Governments have sought to combat discrimination and stigma by providing COVID-19 training to healthcare practitioners. They are using the national press and educational channels to raise public awareness about human rights and underline that the epidemic has no bounds and oppresses people of all ethnicities, faiths, and nationalities. Governments must respect patient confidentiality as authorities attempt to identify individuals who may have been affected by the virus (Human Rights Watch, 2020).

Security for Women

When it comes to women's empowerment, efforts should be increased to determine the crisis's gendered impact. This entails accumulating and analysing current and future sex-disaggregated statistics and data, performing rigorous research, understanding power dynamics at work, personal experiences of various groups, and intersectional components such as ethnicity, caste, class, religion, and others. Assist policymakers, professionals, and non-state leaders in developing accurate, relevant, and timely reaction measures and actions by ensuring widespread data and outcome distribution. Creating a designated receiver for women, as well as other efforts to satisfy the requirements of gender minorities, as well as equal representation of both genders in decision-making and law enforcement. As a result, female farmers, small and medium-sized business owners, and single moms must be prioritized in all transfers, loan programs, and technical support (Rahmadhani et al., 2021).

Fiscal and economic policies are used to address women's economic security by focusing on business operations in sectors with a high percentage of female workers. However, several of them lack essential protection and security measures, such as equitable employment and remuneration: cash transfers, basic food supplies, health insurance, and female-specific social support. They supported pandemic-related government efforts that directly target women, including cash transfers to children and mothers in Myanmar and the Indonesian project Keluarga Harapan, which targets pregnant and breastfeeding women. The bulk of initiatives, particularly in the post-pandemic era, did not develop comprehensive plans for the long-term economic endurance of women. Few governments pandemic-related programmes prioritize women's financial stability. This is especially true in unsavoury female-dominated industries where workers are not protected by labour laws or safety nets and are underpaid, such as manufacturing, clothes (industrial sector), tourism, and catering (services sector). Despite a large number of female service employees, India seemed to have taken the most proactive steps to address this issue.

On the other hand, China, Indonesia, Malaysia, the Philippines, Mongolia, and Thailand have refused to recognize it. In a variety of industries, significant layoffs and furloughs have interrupted female work (Rahmadhani et al., 2021). In Afghanistan, Nepal, Bangladesh, India, and Pakistan, women hold the bulk of agricultural jobs. According to the International Labour Organization (ILO, 2020c), an increase in the number of women working in agriculture represents poverty because it demonstrates a greater gender disparity in employment, high poverty, and lower productivity, with the majority of women performing unpaid labour. Few countries, however, have enacted pandemic-related legislation addressing unpaid labour (Indonesia, China, India, and South Korea, for example).

In reality, it appears that South Korea is the only Asian country with dedicated childcare legislation. Due to a lack of temporary caretakers, the Korean government has set up a number of cash-based programmes to compensate for the transition from daycare to residential care and care for disabled family members. China, India, and Indonesia have all given a variety of social care services for elderly and disabled people, ranging from home-based care to medical support and dietary supplies. While domestic subsidies helped families meet their expenses, there appears to be a lack of direct support or a mechanism in place to support males and females who share parental responsibilities.

According to Rahmadhani et al. (2021), several issues merit addressing, including (1) ensuring that rural women and women from lower-income groups have access to data and information on the measures. (2) Raise public awareness and launch communication initiatives highlighting the need for men to share reproductive responsibility. (3) Ensure that returning labourers are registered with local governments so that they can get social assistance and other forms of help. When migrant workers are subjected to abuse and misinformation, a constructive process for their integration into family and society is triggered. (4) Involve and benefit laid-off people in community programmes, particularly returning foreign workers and other disadvantaged populations. All genders should have an equal opportunity to participate in initiatives and be paid similarly. (5) Form a regional and national network or caucus of female policymakers and formal leaders, as well as female grassroots and grassroots leaders, to conduct research, gather data, and document existing COVID-19 crisis response measures and projects. This codification of women's knowledge can be used as a resource and database for future lessons.

Governments may consider implementing policies to mitigate the economic effects of COVID-19, which will disproportionately harm low-wage workers. Isolation, quarantine, and business closures might all have serious economic consequences. Low-wage workers in low-income households are the most vulnerable. Governments should take steps to prevent COVID-19-infected workers from abandoning their jobs, as this may discourage them from self-isolating in order to keep the virus from spreading. Employers should encourage employees to work from home, according to public health experts. Millions of people working in retail, cafes, the gig economy, professional care, and the informal sector, on the other hand, do not have the option of working remotely. Certain occupations are more volatile, pay less, and in some countries, workers do not receive paid sick leave. These workers require assistance, especially in countries like the United States, where low earnings are combined with a lack of paid medical leave and cheap healthcare. Sick pay and family leave allow employees who are ill—or have a sick family member—to stay at home and prevent disease spread in the case of a COVID-19 epidemic (Human Rights Watch, 2020).

The COVID-19 affects both the supply and demand sides of the labour market, creating major barriers to high employment. More families are falling into poverty as a result of the recession, compounding the existing imbalances (ILO, 2020d). Prudent policymaking and timing are crucial for reducing the financial, employment, and societal effects of the crisis. Immediate stimulus might be required to improve healthcare while reducing the impact on the economy and labour markets. This will be accomplished by providing financial assistance to enterprises (particularly micro and small businesses) and income support to employees. In an ideal scenario, householders would be able to provide immediate and precise estimates of the shutdown's impact on economic activity, employment, and other factors (ILO, 2020e). Prevention of future reductions in investment and consumption is critical. Previous crises have taught us that stimulus packages must include substantial job and social security support.

Workers whose jobs rely on the global economy may be forced to work for less compensation or lose their jobs entirely. One option is to compensate for lost work hours with direct cash payments, as the US government did during the 2008 financial crisis. Low-wage workers must be protected from being fired by their employers because they are unable to work for a lengthy period of time or because a family member is ill. If they do not receive assistance—simple one-time financial awards for families whose children receive free lunch or social security benefits—many workers may suffer significant economic difficulty, default on debt payments, and eviction. Support could help reduce, if not alleviate, the effects on already stressed-out families who may now face new issues, such as school closures, in addition to income loss. Specific government actions are planned or carried out in European countries such as Italy, France, and Spain to aid customers, low-income families, and small businesses.

Employer-side and consumer-side tax cuts are not always properly targeted, and they do not always assist the most vulnerable. Increasing the scope of social insurance programmes such as unemployment insurance could be one of the options. Employees may be allowed to stay principally on payroll and compensated if they

Politics and Electoral System   123

are unable to report to work due to a COVID-19. Many governments offer paid sick leave to all employees. Others, most notably the United States among developed economies, do not. Paid sick leave is unlikely to be accessible to gig economy employees, low-wage earners, service personnel, and informal labourers. Because of a lack of paid sick and family leave, viral illnesses like COVID-19 enhance economic inequality and gender imbalance. Sick and family leave should include self-isolation and caregiver obligations during visits to care and education facilities to assist families during an outbreak (Human Rights Watch, 2020).

Citizen Trust

In the new millennium, public trust in governments and political institutions has declined in both developing and developed countries. One of the most difficult aspects of building citizen trust in government is ensuring that individuals, particularly marginalized communities and the poor, are included in policymaking so that governance becomes representative, participatory, and beneficial to all segments of society. Inadequate governance structures and practices undermine public trust. Intrastate disputes and violence within a country can devastatingly impact regional and global security and peace when governance mechanisms are exclusionary and unavailable key services. In this setting, how to establish trust in government and among socioeconomic actors has become increasingly important in both developed and developing economies (Cheema & Popovski, 2010). The COVID-19 epidemic has thrown a spotlight on the world's leaders' governance and capacity.

In times of calamity, the majority of people naturally seek safety and aid from their governments. When politicians and public servants try to carry out their duties, their credibility and legitimacy swiftly diminish. Emergencies reveal the state of the social contract, and competence is essential in times of crisis (Muggah & Katz, 2020). Under the new social compact, government accountability that prioritizes people and the environment is required. Collective bargaining strives for more equitable income distribution, improved workplace health and safety, a sufficient minimum wage that allows workers to live in dignity, and maximum work hours. The Labour Protection Floor (SPF) is made up of several components, all of which are supported by universal social security. Just transitional efforts to ensure confidence in climate action and necessary corporate vigilance under a UN convention on commerce and human rights are critical for sustaining and rebuilding trust and addressing issues about gender equality. The ILO developed the social protection floor (SPF) approach, drawing on the recent experiences of extending the protection, mostly in developing countries. (…) an integrated set of social policies designed to guarantee income security and access to social services for all, pay particular attention to vulnerable groups and protect and empower people across the life cycle (ILO, 2011).

As the early stages of COVID-19 spread around the world, it is apparent that this disease will not be eradicated. Following these initial waves, epidemiologists anticipate it will erupt in "volcanoes" at various periods and locations, potentially for a long time. It is possible that if vaccinations are discovered, they will not provide lifetime immunity. A single explosion might quickly spread regionally or globally. Because the world cannot remain in a state of constant lockdown, collaboration, knowledge sharing, and obtaining universal health access are the only feasible options (Burrow, 2020). The public good of trust is finite and fleeting. Persuading people to comprehend and accept reason and science requires time and effort. This lengthy process of restoring public trust must begin immediately if governments implement the economic and socio-political adjustments required to create a modern order and tackle climate change. Further deterioration in trust could have fatal effects (Mohan, 2020a, 2020b).

The Future Globalization

How long will countries keep their borders closed? Will these physical borders become commercial borders, and will more countries try to limit commerce production within their own borders (Ullah, Haji-Othman & Daud, 2021)? No one has a definitive answer. Personal protective equipment and ventilators, for example, are in short supply, spurring calls for change. We have heard calls for the reintroduction of domestic manufacturing and the renationalization of critical industries (Pearson, 2020). The idea that businesses and their products should be treated equally regardless of where they come from is under attack. If these and other notions proliferate, the business will be stifled. Countries will lose connectedness, and the commercial pillars to which we have grown accustomed will begin to creak and crumble. The world's degree of global connectedness is predicted to decline in 2020 as a result of the COVID-19 pandemic, but it is unlikely to fall below the 2008–2009 levels. Given the scope of the pandemic, this exceptional resilience is noteworthy in and of itself (Pearson, 2020).

After about two years of the epidemic, popular wisdom believes that globalization is regressing. COVID's rapid spread revealed the contagious risks inherent in a mobile world. Supply systems were interrupted, countries were put on lockdown, and a new brand of nationalism emerged, reshaping global politics (Rippert, 2021). Another takeaway from the crisis is how deeply established globalization is in our economic and cultural DNA. Because of international collaboration, scientists were able to develop medications and vaccines at a rate never before seen in human history (Ullah, 2016; Kaur et al., 2021). While we hunker down in our own countries, international internet traffic grew dramatically, and commerce and finance flow recovered faster than expected. And, despite severe production and shipping disruptions, we should take a moment to appreciate how incredibly well global trade has continued to function (Rippert, 2021).

Rather than retreating, the global economy is entering a new phase, according to Accenture's first Business Futures research, which will dramatically alter the way globalization appears in 2019. By separating the concept of place from worldwide experiences, the pandemic has radically transformed our sense of "where"—both socially and commercially (Rippert, 2021). After more than a year of the pandemic, and with all of its effects on public health, the economy, and all other aspects of society and politics still being reviewed and quantified, it appears appropriate to discuss the pandemic's overall ramifications, particularly for globalization processes. Some argue that globalization cannot be blamed for the virus's uncontrollable spread over the world, though it undoubtedly contributed to the disease's rapid global proliferation. Globalization emerged as a result of technological advancements, the removal of travel restrictions, and the ability of economic players to serve global markets (Cizelj, 2021). At the same time, it should be emphasized that proponents of globalization—while retaining the right to critique some of its worst manifestations—appear to outnumber opponents by a wide margin. It is far more of a question of how to globalize than of whether to do so.

As we have seen, globalization has caused a host of issues, ranging from encouraging economic disparity between the affluent and poor in the global community to allowing the world's most powerful economic players to abuse everyone who lacked protection behind national borders. Simultaneously, deglobalization will almost definitely impede economic expansion—particularly in smaller economies—adversely affecting all sectors of society (Cizelj, 2021; Ullah & Ming Yit Ho, 2021). Globalization has a Janus face, which is both lovely and awful (Eden et al., 2001). Others who support it claim that the benefits outweigh the drawbacks, while those who oppose it want to improve global trade conditions or, in some cases, reverse globalization—GLO (Josephson et al., 2018). As a global tsunami or snow avalanche, GLO can't be stopped but can be swum alongside in the hope of survival for those who are brave enough. In other words, the consequences are determined by human-created policies. As a global economic and political crisis, some perceive the outbreak as a catastrophe. Others feel that, despite the shifting roles of the United States and China in the global community, the fundamental principles of the international order will remain largely unchanged (Cizelj, 2021).

COVID-19 has had an impact on a number of key globalization processes. The most significant change is a paradigm shift in how people understand global supply chains. The disruption of supplier connections caused by this issue, combined with growing worry about over-reliance on China-based distribution networks, has already begun to move government and industry calculations away from efficiency and toward resilience. When supply networks get clogged, components are unable to pass through manufacturing and assembly processes, resulting in lower output. Managing this resilience requires optimizing component stockpiles. Keeping more than necessary incurs additional costs. Inadequate storage exposed manufacturing to supply-chain risks such as missed product sales and angered customers, putting long-term market share at risk. To ensure the durability of supply networks, cost and efficiency need to be balanced. Furthermore, the epidemic is expanding the list of industries deemed important for national security.

High-tech items have been classed in this manner as a result of the recent significant deterioration in US–China relations. COVID-19 is heightening bilateral tensions, raising the prospect of the globe adopting two alternative sets of technology, surveillance, or data filtering and gathering standards: one for advanced industrial nations and another for China and a large proportion, if not all, poor countries. COVID-19 is likely to broaden the definition of "strategic" to include medications, medical supplies, and high-tech products. This could lead to higher tariffs, legislative incentives for capital repatriation, and government subsidies for domestic producers. All of this will strangle the type of free-wheeling globalization that has characterized the last few decades (Gordon, 2020). Regardless of the political demands for decoupling, dividing the global economy into US and Chinese ecosystems will stymie global progress by lowering economies of scale, increasing costs, and fragmenting innovation potential. The fight for supremacy in setting technology standards between China, the United States, and its allies exemplifies the world's division. Governments are acquiring more influence over national data as a result of a growing knowledge of the nexus between technology and political power.

As a result, businesses will increasingly be required to navigate varied value chains and manufacturing standards. While Sino-US ties may set the tone for global geopolitics, the outbreak and its aftermath highlight middle-income countries' necessity to work together as global balancers. As the intermediate state with the most economic clout, Japan also made substantial contributions to the maintenance of international order through coalition formation. Smaller countries want to avoid having to choose between the United States and China. Any such call for middle powers, on the other hand, carries a sense of immediacy. Regardless of the outbreak, the global economy will undergo a dramatic concentration shift during the next few decades. Each of the world's three largest economies—China, the United States, and India—will be larger than the next five combined by 2050. As a result, the window of opportunity for middle-power efficiency is fast closing (Ward, 2020).

Ullah et al. (2020) came to a different conclusion, claiming that there are several possible causes for the likely slowing of economic growth as a result of COVID-19. Reduced commerce, travel, business, and pollution are all factors in systemic climate change. Furthermore, the market will grab the opportunity to build even more advanced technologies for virtual communication and meeting participation. Using Uganda as an example, Igoye (2020) suggested that COVID-19 is unlikely to go away very soon and will not be the last global health pandemic. We should be better prepared for the next pandemic and when people resume movement, migration, and travel.

While Europe struggles to restrict COVID-19's spread and deal with the economic, social, and political ramifications, the outbreak has only recently begun in a number of vulnerable countries. Despite the fact that much ink has been spilled speculating on the consequences of this unprecedented global calamity, its scope, duration, and severity remain largely unknown. What is certain is that the virus poses a substantial risk of wreaking havoc in volatile and conflict-affected areas. While the first goal of European governments should be to rescue their own lives and livelihoods, greater economic and political attention should be paid to individuals living in nations already experiencing conflict and where peace and security are at stake.

Failure to promote the viral response could have far-reaching and devastating consequences in unstable and conflict-torn regions. The virus is leading to aggravating joblessness, food insecurity, resource shortages, marginalization, displacement, and opportunistic actions by radicals, warlords, and even governments. All of the outcomes are likely because of the pandemic: widespread dissatisfaction, postponement of elections and constitutional processes, political instability, and increased insecurity. Political upheaval and rising insecurity will have far-reaching effects on the world peace. Failure to contain the pandemic and its possible or likely consequences, such as population movement, a resurgence of illicit economic activity, and an increase in violence, with women and girls bearing the brunt, will have an impact on states' ability to relax restrictions and resume trade and economic activity.

It is impossible to overestimate the value of the preventive and early intervention. Building political solidarity with civil society and government officials in affected nations while also investing in a systemic conflict-sensitive response suited to each country's specific circumstances could be one way to contain the conflict during the pandemic. The European Institute of Peace is (EIP) assessing COVID-19's impact on the fragile and conflict-affected states in which it operates. The Institute is concentrating on the impact on conflict resolution, peace processes, and agreements and crucial components to watch in the future. While the situation is rapidly shifting, a number of recommendations are developing for European and global bodies tasked with settling questions of peace and conflict during these unprecedented times (EIP, 2020).

The Health Care System

In the wake of COVID-19 pandemic, healthcare systems have been forced to reassess their overall preparedness. There has been a lack of consistency in public health surveillance and accessible infrastructure programmes (Kolie et al., 2019; Mattiuzzi & Lippi, 2020). In particular, acute care settings are found to be incapable of coping with sudden or ongoing surges in workload. Health care systems could not keep up with an exponential rise in demand, despite frequent backup plans (Hick et al., 2020; Kandel et al., 2020). If large-scale policy decisions, such as lockdown measures were not made in an "epidemiologically and timely way," it could have a substantial impact on future health care outcome (Carter & May, 2020). Since healthcare issues in a country should be regarded both internal and possibly global, especially in the case of contagious diseases, the latter is crucial (Ravi et al., 2019). It was also overestimated how quickly the financial impact of a worldwide public health emergency spread to many different sectors of the economy (Rodrguez-Morales et al., 2020).

During the COVID-19 pandemic, public health policy reforms were accelerated and adopted more quickly. There is a shift to a more preventative approach to health care, as well as a major reliance on technology in this new form of healthcare delivery. Constant technological challenges connected to laboratory testing surge capacity, rapid adoption of new technologies and mental health problems are juxtaposed with worries about the preservation of privacy and personal data in times of disaster.

However, despite the COVID-19 outbreak's acceleration of several of the aforementioned processes, such as certification, licensing and reimbursement, there are still numerous concerns that need to be worked out, including technological, privacy and safety issues and lawsuits (Alami et al., 2017; Donaghy et al., 2019). In the context of ethics and individual privacy, the collection and availability of massive amounts of data about people (e.g., via geo-tagged social networks) render complete data anonymization ineffective at protecting the identity of the data source, making it only more difficult but still possible, to (re)identify individuals through the use of advanced systems and triangulation (Cecaj et al., 2016). This means that maintaining openness about the risks of downstream data linking and unintentional human identity theft is an ethical requirement (Garattini et al., 2019). To protect data providers, some systems may function badly if they rely solely on anonymous data, which may threaten information accountability and transparency in the population. Anonymity is considered the ideal practice in today's world, especially during humanitarian crises and epidemics of contagious diseases; however, it cannot be understood as an ethical panacea (Coltart et al., 2018).

Many healthcare systems in many countries are inadequately prepared to deal with catastrophes like the COVID-19 epidemic. Even in sophisticated economies like the United States or the United Kingdom, or Japan, a lack of emergency healthcare facilities has resulted in business closures that could have been averted if proper treatment options had been in place. The topic of public health will be brought up again in the United States (most likely to an Obamacare reform). Simultaneously, in a number of other nations, such as Europe, where the healthcare system is already in place, the emphasis will move to budget prioritizing, as scarcity reduction has frequently resulted in cuts to education and healthcare systems in recent years. It is costly to keep economies from collapsing. As we recover from this disaster, governments around the world will need to figure out how to create and sustain healthcare systems capable of coping with the next pandemic (if any) without shutting down the economy for extended periods of time (Dauba-Pantanacce, 2020). Governments should ensure that all citizens have access to a high-quality healthcare system that is cost-effective, ethical, and culturally relevant. Governments should ensure that health professionals are safeguarded and that social welfare programmes for the families of workers who die or get ill as a result of their employment are in place. Informal labourers, who make up a large percentage of the caregiving business, are included in these initiatives. In previous outbreaks, attacks against healthcare workers were driven by a fear of being covered. Governments should be on the alert for such attacks to deter them and ensure that if they do, they can respond promptly, efficiently, and ethically (Human Rights Watch, 2020).

Governments should use public messaging campaigns to guarantee that virtually all COVID-19-related health services are offered without discrimination, including on the basis of gender or sexual orientation, and that everyone has the right to health care. Governments must take steps to create barriers between health practitioners and illegal migrants, especially in the context of COVID-19 testing or therapy, to ensure that vulnerable people seeking lifesaving care are not subjected to reprisal or deportation. Financial barriers, some governments argue, should not prohibit people from getting COVID-19 testing, treatment, or care. Twenty-eight million individuals in the United States do not have health insurance and roughly a quarter of those who do have coverage face difficulties accessing treatment (Human Rights Watch, 2020). Many people in the United States claim that the high cost of medical care and prescription medications is causing their health to deteriorate. Avoiding medical attention during an outbreak harms the sick people and hastens the spread of the coronavirus. Because citizens are unable to access proper medical care, all governments commit to ensuring that a serious public health crisis does not deteriorate into a human rights disaster. Governments must take steps to ensure that everyone has access to affordable medical care and treatment.

Education and Digitalization

One of the key concerns was how the virus would affect the educational system during the pandemic. Most educational counsellors never considered incorporating a pandemic plan into their strategy, leaving them unprepared for what happened in 2020 and 2021. When the pandemic was first declared, travel restrictions were imposed, students were ordered to return home, number of instructors was reduced, and almost everyone was ordered to begin their online learning. The United Nations conducted a survey of 424 institutions worldwide and discovered that 67% of institution-based learning had been replaced by online learning, and 24% had temporarily ceased most learning (United Nations, 2020). While it may appear that educational life would never be the same, this may not be the case.

The global impact of COVID-19 is diverse and visible in almost every field, most notably health, economics, and education. Since the virus was declared a pandemic in March 2020, there have been numerous daily reports on the virus's impact on the lives of millions of people around the world. As a result, each country's primary priority has switched to restricting the virus's spread and mitigating its impact on society in general and particularly on the most vulnerable communities (Osman, 2020). A global pandemic is not a permanent scenario; over time, institutions will devise a mechanism for safely reintegrating kids into their schools in order for them to complete their education. More than 1.5 billion children (United Nations, 2020) are at risk of falling behind due to school closures (UNICEF, 2020).

However, many children around the world, particularly those from low-income households, do not have access to the internet, personal computers, televisions, or even radios at home, increasing already-existing learning inequities. Students who lack access to the resources needed for home-based learning have fewer options for furthering their education. As a result, many people face the prospect of never returning to school, destroying years of educational success around the world (Human Rights Watch, 2021a, 2021b). With school closures in 188 countries (as of April

2020), many people are looking for new ways to give continued education via technologies such as the Internet, television, and radio. However, access to these technologies is limited in many low- and middle-income countries, particularly among impoverished households.

While more than 90% of countries have policies in place for digital and/or broadcast remote learning, just 60% have done so for pre-primary education (UNICEF, 2020). Government strategies that ensure learning continuity through broadcast or digital media have the ability to reach 69% (at most) of children in pre-primary to secondary school worldwide. Remote learning policies based on broadcast and the Internet are unable to reach 31% of kids (463 million) worldwide (Human Rights Watch, 2021a, 2021b), either due to a lack of adequate technology at home or because the enacted rules did not target them. With 83% of countries using this technique, governments used online platforms to provide education while schools were closed. However, barely one-fourth of the world's schoolchildren were reached. Television has the greatest potential to reach students all across the world (62%). Only 16% of students worldwide may benefit from radio-based learning. Globally, three out of every four students who are not reached by distance learning programmes come from rural areas and/or from low-income families. Given these findings, it is vital that governments should not rely solely on a single distant learning channel to reach all students. Improving access to the Internet and other digital solutions for all children would be a long-term focus to reduce learning hazards (Human Rights Watch, 2021a, 2021b; UNICEF, 2020).

The current crisis serves as a sobering reminder of the vital role that public education plays in communities, societies, and individuals' lives. In our minds, we believe that education is a necessity for living a dignified life, and that knowledge serves as a deterrent against social injustice. Once in a generation we have a chance to transform the world and our educational institutions, and we must decide who we want to be in the process. We have unknowingly arrived at a point where reexamining educational objectives and structuring learning is crucial. Human touch and well-being must be prioritized in educational reform. Technology, particularly online technology that enables cross-platform connection, collaboration, and learning, is a critical tool that, rather than being a panacea, serves as a catalyst for innovation and expanded possibilities. We should be more concerned that a shift to distant digital learning will exacerbate disparities between the developing world and the wealthiest regions.

We must ensure that digitalization does not endanger privacy, freedom of expression, or information self-determination and that it does not lead to invasive surveillance. It is a common misconception that online education is the best option for everyone. To defend the right to education in the face of unprecedented conditions caused by the pandemic and establish the confidence required for global collaboration in pooling resources to provide public educational opportunities. All academic stakeholders must ensure that educational opportunities are used solely to further students' interests and talents. It is critical to guard against corruption and prevent educational resources from being seized and redirected for private gain. In times of crisis and instability, we must reconfirm our principles, or we will be at the mercy of popular notions or deceptive ready-made "solutions." Nothing can ever completely replace collaborative work, communal thought, dialogue, and co-creation (UNESCO, 2020). Governments may use mitigating strategies such as engagement with teachers, school personnel, and teachers' unions. Unions and networks to reclaim lost teaching or contact hours, change school calendars and examination dates, and ensure that teachers and administrators are compensated for extra hours worked. Closing elementary and secondary schools may jeopardize efforts to increase school enrolment and retention in countries with a high proportion of out-of-school children.

Governments should make efforts to ensure that compulsory education is followed—and that school reopening is closely monitored. Education officials should focus their efforts on areas where child labour and child marriage are prominent in order to ensure that all children return to school. There are widespread reports that child marriage is on the rise in underdeveloped and developing countries during the pandemic. Furthermore, administrators should work with refugee community members and parent organizations to guarantee that schools, including those for refugee children, use outreach tactics to ensure the return of children who have been separated from their families to the school. School closures without warning may make it more difficult for low-income families to meet basic needs and put food on the table. Administrations should ensure that low-income children who might otherwise be unable to get subsidized meals do so during school closures (Human Rights Watch, 2020).

Interdependence

As a result of the coronavirus outbreak, there are compelling reasons to question globalization. Many countries around the world have come to realize that they are relying too heavily on other countries to supply their own consumer demands and are now battling to do so (Thangavel et al., 2021). When the virus made its way to the United States, researchers discovered that roughly three-quarters of the medicinal chemicals in that country came from overseas. This percentage is significantly high for antibiotic components (Fontaine, 2020). In addition, many industrialized countries reaped little to no benefit from globalization. Global value chains (GVCs), particularly those controlled by China, are causing many people to reject globalization because of its hazards. Protectionism and self-sufficiency were advocated upon national leaders as a logical next step. As an example, India's Prime Minister Narendra Modi has launched the 'Atmanirbhar Bharat Abhiyan' (Self-Sufficiency in India). EU Commission president Urusula von der Leyen also wants to reduce the length of global value chains because of the EU's dependence on a few offshore suppliers. Emmanuel Macron has also pushed for economic independence by bringing back medical and high-tech jobs to the country (Du et al., 2020).

In just a few months, Changi Airport's (in Singapore) passenger flow went from 5.9 million to just 25,200, a 99.5% drop (Faiola, 2020). Businesses relying on tourism, travel (aviation), and hotels saw severe layoffs and job losses. Many may not return to full capacity for a long time (Thangavel et al., 2021). PPE, ventilators, and generic pharmaceuticals were in high demand when the COVID-19 virus spread around the world. Every nation was forced to confront its dependence on China and other foreign suppliers when it was unable to obtain parts from halted factories in China. However, governments and businesses were inspired to become more self-sufficient even after industries reopened following the outbreak, even after supply networks had steadied. The epidemic has led to a surge in anti-globalization attitudes, a decrease in foreign direct investment (FDI), and a decrease in global commerce. As a result of outsourcing production, many Western and European countries promised to bring back the jobs they lost (Thangavel et al., 2021).

The pandemic has spurred populism and intolerance, putting nations' ability to lead and participate in global institutions in jeopardy. In many countries, populism in political leadership and the global arena has been severely destroyed, not just in their own governments' ability to respond to the pandemic but also in their respective governments' ability to adapt to the pandemic. Increased national debate and social contact between states would completely reveal the epidemic's international political tensions. Despite the fact that the epidemic changed modes of communication, diplomatic acts remained unchanged. The pandemic response, which explains the rationale and ramifications of policy and conduct during a crisis, becomes a vital battleground for global discourse about supremacy, smooth competition, and even the future evaluation of a political structure. States that are better prepared to cope with the problem will have a stronger presence.

On the other hand, others will seek to undercut others' successes by avoiding accountability and politicizing the pandemic through a shift in narrative orientations and amplification of narrative methods. There is no need to divide the world into two camps: Eastern autocracy and Western democracy, in order to find practical solutions to this issue. State competence, in particular public interest in their government, is more important than regime type when it comes to performance. The microscopic ideas of "East–West" and "autocratic-democratic" in traditional international politics should not be used to comprehend the pandemic (Corbett & Veenendaal, 2018). Of course, this does not mean to downplay the democratic principles. Return to reality in terms of major power influence, the speed with which big powers contend, and multipolarization and power rebalancing through global governance will all be trademarks of future foreign policy.

A second aspect of the virus's impact is sociological rather than medical in nature (Ward, 2020). COVID-19 has triggered a surge of xenophobia, which we mentioned earlier, toward internal Chinese migrants, Asian migrants in other countries, and, more lately, European migrants and foreigners in general, including in China and other places where the virus has had an impact. Scapegoating and stigmatization are widespread after natural catastrophes, terrorist attacks, and prior pandemics and epidemics. In general, the pandemic has been exploited to spread anti-migrant propaganda and advocate for stricter immigration controls and fewer rights for migrants. In many countries, newly emerging xenophobia has largely replicated pre-existing discriminatory practices, frequently targeting migrants from areas where COVID-19 infection is rare or non-existent, as well as people who have resided in the country for a long time.

The Gainers and the Losers

As a result of COVID-19, billions of people around the world have been suffering from debilitating effects on their health and livelihoods. As COVID-19 continues to shake health, economic, and social systems around the world, governments and development finance institutions have rushed out rescue packages and large-scale initiatives to restore workers and livelihoods. According to Abay and colleagues (2020), demand for some services soared while demand for others decreased drastically as a result of the outbreak. In determining the losers and winners, they considered demand and supply. While demand for services requiring face-to-face encounters decreased significantly as the pandemic progressed, demand for services needing less in-person engagement surged (Abay et al., 2020).

Kelly (2020) argues that since millions of individuals now work from home and spend the majority of their hours there, it's no surprise that millions of people are considering home improvements. Computers, internet, workstations, chairs, and software, as well as anything else that will make working with clients, coworkers, and supervisors simpler online, are all on their shopping list (Kelly, 2020), and hence this rapidly expanding trend benefits companies (such as Google, Microsoft, Amazon, and Best Buy) that provide these goods and services considerably. Kelly (2020) goes on to say that reduced commuting means fewer cars and buses on the road. Since we save money on gas as a result of this, Airline operators have already declared that they will be unable to fly for the time being, and that about 90% flights were grounded. Fear of a COVID-19 revival will force families to avoid flying. Russia and Saudi Arabia are already engaged in a pricing war, which is negatively impacting the oil industry, which is already seeing lower global demand due to the suspension of operations across the globe caused by this trend (Kelly, 2020).

Thakur (2020) made some well-informed predictions on who will win and lose. It is Thakur's opinion that the United States will suffer the most as a result of this. Thakur says the US followed China's original script of denials, cover-ups, and blame-shifting without seeing the irony. The disease has the potential to harm America's economic and moral standing as a world leader. Concerns about the United States' ability to respond effectively to the world's ever-increasing issues had already been raised by President Trump's extraordinary display of incompetence, recklessness, and self-absorption (Thakur, 2020). The race will be won by China, according to Thakur (2020). The EU wasted a once-in-a-generation opportunity. The bulk of countries opted to fight a shared enemy on their own rather than unite to do so. It was shown that certain countries were unwilling to share the borrowing expenses to support the most vulnerable members, reinforcing north–south tensions and prejudices.

President Trump has repeatedly voiced his displeasure over the Atlantic partnership. Europeans have become increasingly distrustful of the United States when it comes to integrity and common sense. With unprecedented state power expansion, even during wartime, supported by big technology persecution of skeptics and dissenting opinions repression, the liberal component of democracy's basic philosophy has been badly undermined. According to Thakur, the East Asian model of competence, superb leadership, and social capital will triumph over all others. The inherent advantages of Japan, Taiwan, South Korea, Vietnam, and Singapore included high-quality health governance, societal cohesion, trust in public institutions, and a willingness to learn and correct past mistakes (Thakur, 2020).

Compared to Europe, the Asian population is more submissive and less dissatisfied (Wintour, 2020). Generally, they have more faith in the government, sometimes without any reason though. Asians have a strong focus on digital surveillance to prevent the spread of the virus. Aside from virologists and epidemiologists, computer scientists and big data experts in Asia are helping to fight disease (Wintour, 2020). If the epidemic has deteriorated into a global leadership contest, countries that respond to the crisis most effectively will rise to the top of the world stage. Their countries' handling of the problem is defended by diplomats who work in decommissioned embassies and take offence when they are called out for their actions (Wintour, 2020).

Non-COVID-19 patients, according to Sharma and colleagues (2020), have borne the brunt of the gross neglect as their health neared a collapse as a result of surging COVID-19 cases. While women in the workplace and at home (as violence against women has increased), restaurants, higher education, airlines, cruise lines, professional sports, and tourism are considered losers, the housing industry, billionaires appear to be winners. Between April and July 2020, when the crisis reached its zenith, more than two-thirds of the world's wealthiest people boosted their fortunes by more than a quarter (27.5%). During the coronavirus outbreak, the world's billionaires amassed a record $10.2 trillion (£7.8 trillion). According to research, the overwhelming majority of billionaires benefited from betting on the global stock market's March and April comeback. The US Securities and Exchange Commission (US SEC) reported that billionaires' net worth had reached a "new high," surpassing the previous record of $8.9 trillion set in 2017, as a result, the global population of billionaires has increased to 2,189, up from 2,158 in 2017 (Neate, 2020).

Getting Ready for the Future

'With over 273,978,147 recorded infections and nearly 5,360,789 confirmed deaths and 245,847,419 recoveries, COVID-19 is causing the most lethal pandemic since the Spanish Flu of 1918–1920.' More than 0.1% of the world's population has already been lost in a growing number of countries (more than one in a thousand). This includes the United Kingdom (0.12%), but also Belgium (0.18%), Italy (0.13%), Czechia (0.13%), the United States (0.12%), Peru (0.12%), Spain (0.11%), and Mexico (0.11%) (Worldometers, 2021). Given that we have yet to see the first global high, these cases are expected to grow for the foreseeable future (Miller, 2021). Much remains unknown about COVID-19 and its future development. For example, we don't know how long COVID-19 survivors will be protected from re-infection or how long vaccine protection will last and how many boosters we may need. Pfizer's ability to halt Omicron's spread is a questionable conclusion drawn by powerful countries. Doubt looms because it should not have come this quickly. How was that feasible making such inference prior to conducting systematic research? We have no clue how to determine whether or not a person is protected. We do not know how many survivors will acquire 'long COVID' or the full scope of the disorder. We do not know how frequently new variants may emerge or how this will affect our reaction to COVID-19. However, there is light at the end of the tunnel and reason to be optimistic, as vaccines have been made available, though disproportionately, to protect a substantial percentage of people, (Miller, 2021).

As the COVID-19 situation evolves, any estimations or advice regarding the future route of the situation will be imprecise and approximate. Only informed guesses on its size and, more importantly, length are possible. Uncertainties include the severity of the crisis in the industries most affected by the lockdown, the quantity of unemployment, and the extent to which governments will interfere in the economy. It is yet unclear how these and countless other concerns will play out globally or nationally. Failure to maintain global health safety will have far-reaching consequences in politics, economics, and the public realm. Increased pessimism, xenophobia, misinformation, regressive tendencies, a lack of trust at all levels of government, and a distorted economy will need efforts to strengthen international collaboration. Businesses that transport goods and services across national borders and through value-added networks are already feeling the strain.

Notably, the epidemic has played a significant role in escalating tensions between the United States and China. Each of them has remained strong to accuse others of being a threat to humankind as a whole. This dispute jeopardizes economic globalization and stymies efforts to strengthen institutions for long-term development. These characteristics make it more difficult to resurrect institutions that have fallen short of the purpose of putting together a collective response to contemporary challenges. On the other hand, current and prospective hazards are more obvious than ever. Despite the failure of significant powers to demonstrate necessary solidarity, non-state entities can step forward and assume additional responsibility (Yurgens, 2020). According to foresight, policymakers should be informed of critical future changes and have access to policy options. The goal of this analysis is to identify patterns that may have an impact on domestic and international issues. These compass points are the result of the political repercussions of technological breakthroughs such as social media and election manipulation, drones and defence policy, and the continuous monitoring of important governance metrics (such as financial improvement, status, or the increase of illness). Based on how these events and signs are evaluated, policy recommendations define the activities that should be taken to avert an impending crisis or manage an expected danger (Brozus, 2020).

As they confront the ravages of coronavirus, or COVID-19, all governments, provinces, and cities share a sense of foreboding. In light of the pandemic's far-reaching implications for health, the global economy, and global interests and worldviews, the outbreak needs a reassessment of the concept of global unity and the role of global governance. Global and economic crises will need much enhanced international coordination and considerably more active measures to avoid worst-case scenarios. Given the failure of major international political parties to respond to COVID-19, more focus should be placed on more adaptive international technical organizations with the competence, access, and demonstrated ability to respond quickly to emerging events. Given that such institutions are inextricably linked to the political environments in which they emerge and operate, detailed changes to increase openness and construct processes to assure responsibility for crucial decisions are required.

Even while great-power competition is expected to remain a factor in global dynamics for the foreseeable future, such measures would help to limit the risks of the dysfunction represented and reinforced by the current global response to COVID-19 (Hatuel-Radoshitzky & Heistein, 2020). Institutional renewal should be founded on a rethinking of the goals of international politics. Existential risks necessitate a rebalancing of government and policy research. Along with the still-dominant fear of nuclear war and the more recent emphasis on climate change mitigation, biosecurity issues must be elevated to the top of the global agenda. Biosecurity is still a low priority when it comes to threat analysis and forecasting. They rejected official national security documentation from a number of countries. When these issues are discussed in-depth, the tone becomes more declarative and ambiguous in Russia's national security strategy. This implies that breakthroughs in biotechnology can have a mixed impact on regional and global security. As a result, global governance organizations must adopt new policies to limit or prohibit research in specific areas of biotechnology and biomedicine and methods for centralized, agile, and thorough management and verification of the market supply for their products (Yurgens, 2020). The COVID-19 crisis demonstrates the importance of long-term political leadership from the United Nations, development economic institutions, and clubs like the Community of Seven (CoS) and the Group of Twenty (G20) in ensuring a coordinated and successful global response to a global economic crisis. Improved financial coordination, going beyond the current efforts of the IMF and the G20. Flexible finance options to respond quickly to the socioeconomic implications of COVID-19, significantly enhanced technical and economic support for the WHO, and increased intellectual and health collaboration, particularly on vaccines, are all immediate critical components of such a response. Long-term leadership also entails releasing COVID-19 vaccines, medications, and medical equipment from the economic limits imposed by pharmaceutical firms and other manufacturers.

A fresh landscape for development cooperation has emerged in the aftermath of the COVID-19 epidemic. The numerous repercussions of COVID-19 for individuals, groups, and regions, as well as the prospect of aggravated territorial imbalances, necessitate a place-based approach to regional development, improved inclusivity, and a renewed sense of urgency. The value of top-down and bottom-up activity balance, the need for successful connections and trust across numerous groups of actors, the need for adaptability and flexibility, and the importance of top-down and bottom-up activity balance all contribute to this urgency. Furthermore, it has rekindled policy arguments about regional resilience. Local development objectives have altered in favour of regional resilience development as a result of the epidemic's demands on all levels of government (OECD, 2020a). In COVID-19, governments are working in a state of great uncertainty. The COVID-19 problem has numerous local and regional repercussions that are important for problem management and policy involvement. The study investigates the COVID-19 crisis's spatial consequences in all of its dimensions: health, economy, social, and fiscal. It offers examples of regional and national government actions that have contributed to minimizing the crisis's territorial ramifications, as well as a few essential lessons for coping with COVID-19's territorial ramifications (OECD, 2020a). The preceding highlighted challenges do not imply a negative view of global development cooperation. Certain positive traits should be reinforced as well. Countries in Europe with a history of humanism and additive values remain key sponsors of global development aid, as indicated by their support for the WHO and global pandemic prevention measures in the face of COVID-19 (Gilmore et al., 2020). Private organizations, such as the Bill and Melinda Gates Foundation, have also made important contributions to global development, most notably in the areas of global food and health security. Throughout the outbreak, emerging countries increased their aid to developing countries while decreasing aid to developed countries. As a result, the global development assistance system retains critical elements of solidarity. Preliminary research by Zhou et al. (2020) indicates that the post-COVID-19 development partnership will have four crucial characteristics:

The COVID-19 pandemic motivates society to confront the new global crisis, increasing human capacity to address new emerging issues. Because of the epidemic's rapid spread and breadth, fighting together is crucial to engage in comprehensive and innovative development cooperation, whether focusing on capacity building or establishing governance models. Cooperation is currently the only realistic option for common security. The priority of development cooperation will then move to "human security" in the post-pandemic phase. International development assistance has primarily focused on good governance, anti-corruption, and domestic economic growth since the end of the Cold War. The implications of the epidemic have progressively persuaded governments around the world that international cooperation must centre on human security, global health, food security, climate change, governance, and agriculture. A new structural foundation for global prosperity is required to address human security issues. Multilateralism can only benefit all countries if they actively promote, campaign for, and support it, most notably by recognizing the UN's critical role in assisting developing countries, whether developed, emerging, or developing, in overcoming obstacles and progressing toward common and ideal goals (Cheng, 2020; Cotula, 2021).

As a result of the pandemic, numerous governments have launched lockdown measures or adopted a patchwork of regulatory restrictions. However, given the worldwide breadth of the problem and the seriousness of its consequences, these concerns will continue to be crucial for organizations that gather data and promote accountability. A robust research and practice agenda is required to investigate these traits both during and after the pandemic. To address the issue, scholars and practitioners must refrain from local-to-global collaborations while also providing practical avenues for individuals whose rights are most directly at stake to pursue their interests.

Reopening Plans

When the governor of Georgia and other senior officials in the United States advocate for the removal of legislation aimed at preventing the spread of the coronavirus, they, without doubt, put millions of people in danger. There are further non-medical dangers associated with the coronavirus' proliferation. According to the leading epidemiologists and the majority of mainstream economists, there is a possibility that the already severe economic impact will worsen and last longer than we thought. In today's interconnected world, doctors say that the coronavirus's ability to spread is what makes the threats so important (Lee, 2020). Truth be told, the danger to health does not only apply to people who are out and about, instead, it is for everyone else in the community.

When it comes to dealing with an illness, former US President Donald Trump believes that the therapy is riskier. Conservative politicians and economists have recently contributed their voices to the debate with a variety of different viewpoints on the issue (Lee, 2020). Absolutely unethical is how supply-side economist Arthur Laffer described strangling the economy and denying future generations of chances, while Texas Lt. Gov. Dan Patrick remarked that we are smothering the economy. Even economists cannot agree on whether the outbreak is a case of cost–benefit analysis or not. It is not uncommon for corporate leaders and accountants to conduct these kinds of tasks (Lee, 2020). When dealing with the coronavirus, it is difficult to construct an equation since there are so many variables to consider, such as how many people will be infected, how many will get sick or die, and the long-term financial impact.

However, some discussion has taken place on how this trade-off between life and economy should be quantified and addressed. To ensure that all G7 economies can reopen on a solid foundation, the presidents of the G7 countries asked their ministers to work together to ensure that all G7 economies are prepared for safe reopening on the basis of more resilient health systems trustworthy supply networks.

A prolonged lockdown would have a negative impact on both the economy and social structure of countries and regions that had weathered the worst of the pandemic. When it comes to local health and the influence of reopening policies, the issue has risen to the top in municipal as well as in global governments' agendas and on social media. The lack of pandemic models with several epicentres means that simulations cannot be used to help formulate policies during the reopening phase (Zhong, 2021). As the reopening process gains momentum around the world, the most severe test yet is about to arrive for those who have welcomed free borders and mobility to brand themselves as the best spots to be during an epidemic (Bloomberg, 2021).

The United Arab Emirates and Chile have moved up to the top ten of Bloomberg's COVID Resilience Ranking after implementing similar vaccination policies that provide vaccinated individuals greater leeway. It's been another month in the lead for Ireland, despite an increase in accidents. Over 90% of the population has been immunized, and the country is cautiously reopening, allowing pubs and restaurants to resume regular business hours for immunized clients, and that there has been

Getting Ready for the Future

a significant decline in the number of hospitalizations since the pandemic began (Bloomberg, 2021; Brenan, 2021).

Monthly snapshots are provided by the COVID Resilience Ranking, which shows where the virus is being treated most effectively and with the least social and economic impact. Which country has the best and worst response to a once-in-a-generation threat is determined by a ranking of 12 data variables, including viral containment, healthcare quality, vaccine coverage, overall mortality, and progress toward resuming travel (Chang & Tam, 2021). Spain and the United Arab Emirates round out the top three. A summer epidemic of the delta variant in Spain, one of the worst-hit countries at the beginning of the pandemic, saw a decrease in infections, positive testing rates, and mortality. Airplane capacity has returned to pre-COVID levels, while social gathering restrictions have been loosened and curfews have been abolished. As the country prepares to hold the World Expo in Dubai, the UAE has climbed three spots, but it may face extra hazards as new infections fall to their lowest level in more than a year in October 2021 (Bloomberg, 2021; Cornwell, 2021).

If the United States cannot reinvigorate a sluggish vaccination campaign and overcome a relatively high delta death toll, it may face additional pressure. As a result of an increase in fatalities, the United Kingdom slipped nine positions to 25th. For the third month in a row, Indonesia, Malaysia, Thailand, Vietnam, and the Philippines remain in the bottom six of the world's most corrupt countries, which has implications for COVID-19 combat. However, despite recent progress in immunization efforts in Malaysia, many of these export-dependent countries continue to bear the brunt of the delta's impact. However, catching up with Europe and the U.S. will take some time for these countries to get back on their feet (Bloomberg, 2021).

It seems with a full COVID winter upon them, Europe will put its success to the test. There has been a substantial increase in cases in the UK, Belgium, Ireland, and other European countries as a result of the region's pioneering measures of prolonging the time between doses and limiting quarantine-free entrance to persons who have been inoculated (Bloomberg, 2021). As the world's most damaged region, South America, continues to recover, Chile's rapid leap from the bottom half of the ranking to the top eight happened in less than a month. Immunizations have been given to millions, internal restrictions have been relaxed, and overseas tourists subject to a five-day quarantine have been able to travel again. In November, it will be even easier for passengers to go through quarantine (Mega, 2020).

Economists prefer to think of the economy in terms of numbers on a computer screen, but, in fact, the economy is people, Rust (2020) said in response to a question about the impact of COVID-19 on the service sector. We may consider a modest retail shop as an analogy. It is likely that the things it offers bring in a small profit. There are a lot of small-town businesses getting slammed. In many cases, these enterprises lack the financial wherewithal to function without revenue for a long period of time. This is expected to result in the closure of 70% of restaurants. If someone runs a small business, they can take advantage of the Paycheck Protection Programme. However, the distribution of funds has been extremely delayed. As a result, a large number of businesses have received finance from large banks.

Rust (2020) asserts that if small businesses lack the cash to operate, they will not be able to accept social distance, which is another worry. Many of these businesses will never return for business. Amazon, for example, is expected to benefit greatly from this trend, as the retail industry as a whole has been shrinking for some time now due to online purchasing. Pizza delivery services, such as Domino's, will prosper in the future. Online retailers are going to do really well. They are already doing a great job. Grocery stores are also doing well, which is not a surprise given the amount of food Americans eat. There is no doubt that some people will come out on top. The winners are not affected by this situation. The fear is that a large number of people will lose out. If the retail store closes, the employees will no longer be able to contribute to the economy or hire new workers implying that there will be a negative multiplier effect (Rust, 2020).

Some people say that this pandemic has taught us how to be resilient—the ability to cope with adversity and overcome trauma. A once-in-a-lifetime chance to improve our grasp of resilience has been afforded by the epidemic (Pariès, 2020). The announcement by the President of the French Republic in a military operation dubbed Resilience to combat the COVID-19 outbreak causes a concern. Indeed, the pandemic is altering the safety management of high-risk industries. When it comes to productivity, profitability, industrial safety, occupational health and safety and environmental impact, health considerations are taking precedence over these other aspects. The outbreak necessitates a reduction in manpower and a curtailment of on-site activity in the field (Pariès, 2020).

Conclusions

Because the current outbreak will serve as a baseline for future crises of equal proportions, it will underline the critical role of the state in planning and organizing actions to confront global health security risks, whether on a domestic or multilateral scale. The epidemic will exacerbate current political tensions on a societal level by instilling fear in more countries, prompting them to turn to protectionism and nationalistic instincts. Except for growing disparities and a renewed emphasis on pre-pandemic political reasons, no significant new political tools will be generated to respond to the pandemic's ramifications (Aldalala'a, 2020). Financial and commercial concerns will drive geostrategic and global politics. The current disruption differs from previous shocks in its abruptness, global impact, and unpredictability of recovery. Furthermore, it takes up space at a time when global power is at stake. The global supply chain has been re-examined as a result of a convergence of factors, and significant vulnerabilities have been uncovered.

A shift toward a more locally based global economy may help counterbalance rising populism, nationalism, and protectionism by creating a more balanced connection between domestic and international concerns. While future technologies may improve resilience and efficiency, regionalization may have a negative impact on global well-being by limiting the scale and raising prices. Given the expected loss

Conclusions 141

of intergovernmental expertise and FDI flows, the FDI repercussions are significant. Intraregional flows, on the other hand, have increased. While global value chains (GVCs) are projected to reduce in size, fragmentation will occur as intraregional specialization grows. Regional growth will be stimulated by reshoring and nearshoring in existing centres such as the United States, China, and Germany. As regional specialization expands, investments will become more market-driven than efficiency-driven.

Vertical FDI will be bolstered by growing horizontal investment as areas seek to diversify their talent pools. In order to avoid unnecessary duplication, increased competition for FDI will necessitate strong regional coordination, investment promotion, and industrial policy. The intraregional collaboration will become increasingly important as global specialization gives way to regional specialization. Finally, the efficiency costs of further regionalization must be balanced against the potential for constructing a more inclusive, egalitarian, and acceptable global governance (Enderwick & Buckley, 2020). Today's predicament is more than just redoubling our efforts to safeguard democracy. A more thorough review is essential due to the epidemic's potential to alter several democratic processes. The post-pandemic development strategy needs prioritize strategic an in-depth study of the current crisis's lessons. The COVID-19 epidemic exposed a lack of preparedness in a number of countries throughout the world. Planning is a democratic duty that allows for deliberate reactions while reducing panic. As a result, a greater emphasis on foresight in crisis management is required to limit the detrimental impact of random acts on democracy (Youngs & Panchulidze, 2020).

The advent of COVID-19, or at least its second phase in several nations, has stressed the significance of multi-level governance, as well as a place-based approach to crisis response and restoration. The importance of strong leadership with effective collaboration and consulting, as well as the benefits of centrally managed versus decentralized crisis management, are discussed in greater depth. There needs to be public trust, not just in crisis management but also in health outcomes, and good communication between internal and external stakeholders. Because of this, countries are being forced to put more emphasis on rural development as an approach to increasing survival by ensuring that people everywhere have equal access to essential services, closing digital gaps, achieving net zero emissions, and making the most of the opportunities that globalization presents them with. The impact of COVID-19 on communities, counties, and countries has prompted a broader discussion about resilience and preparing for future health, financial, and social crises (OECD, 2020a, 2020b). As the year comes to a close, there is still a lot of doubt regarding the path of COVID-19, but there is a growing consensus that the disease will be around for at least another two years. Vaccines being more widely available in 2021, on the other hand, will pave the way for improved disease control. Even if this were true, the pandemic's political tensions would continue to ripple over the world, especially given the expected uneven and delayed nature of the global economic recovery.

It will take years for the global travel and tourism industry to recover the loss incurred. Reviving the informal economy in the world's two most populous countries, China and India, which account for the majority of each country's employment, would present significant obstacles. Both the US and China's image in global geopolitics have been harmed. It was the result of the United States' failure to curb the virus, as well as China's exaggeration of its influence in international affairs. On the other hand, Europe has become stronger, but its contributor, German Chancellor Angela Merkel, will step aside in 2021. Her performance on the European stage will be difficult to replicate as well. COVID-19 will loom large over global politics, increasing hurdles and fostering mistrust. However, it will provide incentives and chances for countries to look past their differences in order to achieve common health, economic, and security goals (Gordon, 2020).

According to the IOM, migrants, like many other citizens, share these vulnerabilities and the difficulties that come with them (IOM, 2021). While the IOM focuses on people who have been forced to relocate, its issues also apply to migrant labourers. Internally Displaced Persons (IDPs), including those in camps and those living in non-camp settings and slum dwellers and the impoverished, may experience the same social distance and hygienic restrictions as migrant workers. Workers in the gig or informal economy are more likely to lose their jobs if their employers or the government do not support them. Meanwhile, those from impoverished and marginalized groups will have restricted access to health care (IOM, 2021: 4). COVID-19's impact varies according to migrants' and residents' socioeconomic circumstances: in the United Kingdom, ethnic minorities were rapidly identified as being overrepresented among those most likely to die from COVID-19, notably among National Health Service staff.

Is the COVID-19 outbreak likely to reignite nationalism? What effect will the present global revival of nationalist populism have on the pandemic's response? The primary issue is whether COVID-19 will intensify nationalism and ethnic conflict and how this will affect the possibilities for nation-building. At the time of writing, we are still in the third phases of the pandemic, when even the most basic terms of reference are difficult to grasp and fast-changing. We believe that historical and theoretical reflection can help recognize emergent trends despite these challenges.

We must determine our political stance on the COVID-19 epidemic. Despite the pandemic being frequently referred to as a "crisis," more information in this area can help us map COVID-19's potential political implications. Actual or imagined hazards precipitate crises. They are severely disruptive events that add to uncertainty (by disrupting plans, routines, expectations, beliefs, and values) (Brecher et al., 2021; Quarantelli & Dynes, 1977; Rosenthal et al., 1989). This instability and unpredictability have the potential to change the political situation (Falleti & Lynch, 2009). External shocks that cause structural indeterminacy frequently trigger these transitions, which are referred to as "critical junctures" (Capoccia & Kelemen, 2007; Falleti & Lynch, 2009; Mahoney, 2001).

Pandemic fears have already triggered a chain reaction of health and economic concerns, and they now threaten to engulf politics and upend the nationalist milieu in which most international politics is conducted (Woods et al., 2020). There are a few fallacies about COVID-19 and vaccines. Is it true that the COVID-19 vaccines result in infertility in their recipients? This argument serves as a red herring, deflecting attention away from the essential subject. In this scenario, the Bill Gates lawsuits and

Conclusions   143

information suppression divert attention away from the core worry that COVID-19 vaccinations induce infertility. Concentrating on the vaccine's safety rather than on side issues such as online information and lawsuits is critical for resolving this worry. According to some, vaccines may trigger autoimmune disorders (Smith, 2021). Vaccines are unlikely to cause autoimmunity since, in general, they cannot cause something that a disease cannot, such as autoimmune illness. The vaccination is unlikely to produce autoimmunity, as COVID-19 patients do not develop autoimmune diseases. Long-term adverse effects of this vaccination have been heard. This is an instance of an appeal to ignorance, as it is centred on the unknown. To arouse doubt, the concept of COVID-19 vaccinations has been used to assert that we do not know what would happen years after vaccination. While ignorance is a lethal weapon, it is critical to maintain a focus on the truth. We know that COVID-19 vaccinations are rapidly digested and do not persist in the body for an extended period of time (Children's Hospital Philadelphia, 2021). When there is an emergency, the policy should take precedence over politics. In truth, natural disasters exacerbate underlying flaws in political and economic processes, such as elite distrust.

References

Abay, K. A., Tafere, K., & Woldemichael, A. (2020). *Winners and losers from COVID-19: Global evidence from Google Search* (World Bank Policy Research Working Paper No. 9268). Retrieved from: https://openknowledge.worldbank.org/handle/10986/33852. License: CC BY 3.0 IGO.

Alami, H., Gagnon, M. P., Wootton, R., Fortin, J. P., & Zanaboni, P. (2017). Exploring factors associated with the uneven utilization of telemedicine in Norway: A mixed methods study. *BMC Medical Informatics and Decision Making, 17*(1), 1–15.

Aldalala'a, N. (2020, April 23). The impact of Covid-19 on global politics: 'It is all in the response'. *Trends*. Retrieved from: https://trendsresearch.org/insight/the-impact-of-covid-19-on-global-politics-it-is-all-in-the-response/. Accessed 30 July 2021.

Aldrich, J. H. (1993). Rational choice and turnout. *American Journal of Political Science, 37*(1), 246–278.

Anadolu Agency. (2020). *COVID-19: Some 4.5M African jobs to be lost in 2020*. Retrieved from: https://www.aa.com.tr/en/africa/covid-19-some-45m-african-jobs-to-be-lost-in-2020/1992666

Asian Development Bank. (2021a). *The effect of COVID-19 on foreign direct investment*. https://www.adb.org/publications/effect-covid-19-foreign-direct-investment

Asian Development Bank. (2021b). *Key indicators for Asia and the Pacific 2021*.

Ayittey, F. K., Ayittey, M. K., Chiwero, N. B., Kamasah, J. S., & Dzuvor, C. (2020). Economic impacts of Wuhan 2019-nCoV on China and the world. *Journal of Medical Virology, 92*(5), 473–475.

Ball, M. (2020a, October 8). Donald Trump's COVID-19 diagnosis is forcing him to face his personal—And political—Vulnerability. *Time*. Retrieved from: https://time.com/5897886/trump-coronavirus/. Accessed 30 July 2021.

Ball, M. (2020b, August 6). How COVID-19 changed everything about the 2020 election. Retrieved from: https://time.com/5876599/election-2020-coronavirus/. Accessed 29 July 2021.

Benzian, H., Beltran-Aguilar, E., Mathur, M. R., & Niederman, R. (2021). Pandemic considerations on essential oral health care. *Journal of Dental Research, 100*(3), 221–225.

Bhanot, D., Singh, T., Verma, S. K.,& Sharad, S. (2021). Stigma and discrimination during COVID-19 pandemic. *Frontiers in Public Health, 829*. https://doi.org/10.3389/fpubh.2020.577018

Black, R., Natali, C., & Skinner, J. (2005). Migration and inequality. *World Bank*. Retrieved from: https://openknowledge.worldbank.org/handle/10986/9172. Accessed 4 Aug 2021.

Bloomberg. (2021, November 30). *The Covid resilience ranking*. Retrieved from: https://www.bloomberg.com/graphics/covid-resilience-ranking/. Accessed 15 July 2021.

BRAC Institute of Governance and Development (BIGD). (2020). Trust, institutions, and collective action rapid study of community responses to Covid-19 in Bangladesh. *Policy Brief.* BRAC Institute of Governance and Development.

Bradford, C. I. (2020, September 24). *Global goals and domestic politics: The missing connective tissue is now palpably present*. Retrieved from: https://www.brookings.edu/opinions/global-goals-and-domestic-politics-the-missing-connective-tissue-is-now-palpably-present/. Accessed 09 July 2021.

Brecher, E. A., Keels, M. A., Carrico, C. K., & Hamilton, D. S. (2021, Nov 15). Teledentistry implementation in a private pediatric dental practice during the COVID-19 pandemic. *Pediatric Dentistry, 43*(6), 463–467. PMID: 34937617.

Brenan, M. (2021, November 16). Roundup of Gallup COVID-19 Coverage. *GALLUP*. Retrieved from: https://news.gallup.com/opinion/gallup/308126/roundup-gallup-covid-coverage.aspx. Accessed 24 Nov 2021.

Brown, F. Z., Brechenmacher, S., & Carothers, T. (2020, April 06). How will the coronavirus reshape democracy and governance globally? *Carnegie Endowment for International Peace*. Retrieved from: https://carnegieendowment.org/2020/04/06/how-will-coronavirus-reshape-democracy-and-governance-globally-pub-81470. Accessed 30 July 2021

Brozus, L. (2020). The difficulty of anticipating global challenges: The lessons of COVID-19. In T. Bernes, L. Brozus, M. Hatuel-radoshitzky, A. Heistein, E. Greco et al. (Eds.), *Challenges of global governance amid the COVID-19 pandemic* (pp. 6–9). Council on Foreign Relations: International Institutions and Global Governance Program.

Burrow, S. (2020). Work: The pandemic that stopped the world. In *World economic forum*. http://www3.weforum.org/docs/WEF_Challenges_and_Opportunities_Post_COVID_19.pdf. Accessed 30 July 2021.

Capoccia, G., & Kelemen, R. (2007). The study of critical junctures: Theory, narrative, and counterfactuals in historical institutionalism. *World Politics, 59*(3), 341–369. https://doi.org/10.1017/S0043887100020852

Carter, D. P., & May, P. J. (2020). Making sense of the US COVID-19 pandemic response: A policy regime perspective. *Administrative Theory & Praxis, 42*(2), 265–277.

Cassella, M. (2020). *A growing side effect of the pandemic: Permanent job loss*. Retrieved from: https://www.politico.com/news/2020/08/06/coronavirus-permanent-unemployment-392022

Cecaj, A., Mamei, M., & Zambonelli, F. (2016). Re-identification and information fusion between anonymized CDR and social network data. *Journal of Ambient Intelligence and Humanized Computing, 7*(1), 83–96.

Chang, R., & Tam, F. (2021). *Methodology: Inside Bloomberg's Covid resilience ranking*. Retrieved from: https://financialpost.com/pmn/business-pmn/methodology-inside-bloombergs-covid-resilience-ranking-2. Accessed 22 Dec 2021.

Cheema, G. S., & Popovski, V. (Eds.). (2010). *Building trust in government: Innovations in governance reform in Asia* (Vol. 139). United Nations University Press.

Cheng, M. (2020). The impact of COVID-19 on patterns of international relations and the world order. *The Dig*. https://thedig.nz/transitional-diplomacy/the-impact-of-covid-19-on-patterns-of-international-relations-and-the-world-order/. Accessed 30 July 2021.

Children's Hospital Philadelphia. (2021). News & views—Name the logical fallacy: COVID-19 edition. Retrieved from: https://www.chop.edu/news/news-views-name-logical-fallacy-covid-19-edition. Accessed 22 Dec 2021.

Cizelj, B. (2021). *The impact of Covid-19 on the future globalisation*. Retrieved from: https://wsimag.com/economy-and-politics/65858-the-impact-of-covid-19-on-the-future-globalisation

Coltart, C. E. M., Hoppe, A., Parker, M., Dawson, L., Amon, J. J., Simwinga, M., Geller, G., Henderson, G., Laeyendecker, O., Tucker, J. D., Eba, P., Novitsky, V., Vandamme, A. M., Seeley,

References

J., Dallabetta, G., Harling, G., Grabowski, M. K., Godfrey-Faussett, P., Fraser, C., Cohen, M. S., Pillay, D. (2018, Nov). Ethics in HIV phylogenetics working group. Ethical considerations in global HIV phylogenetic research. *Lancet HIV, 5*(11), e656–e666. https://doi.org/10.1016/S2352-3018(18)30134-6. Epub 2018 Aug 30. PMID: 30174214; PMCID: PMC7327184.

Converse, P. E. (2000). Assessing the capacity of mass electorates. *Annual Review of Political Science, 3*(1), 331–353.

Coppedge, M., Gerring, J., Altman, D., Bernhard, M., Fish, S., Hicken, A., Kroenig, M., Lindberg, S. I., McMann, K., Paxton, P., Semetko, H. A., Skaaning, S.-E., Staton, J., & Teorell, J. (2011). Conceptualizing and measuring democracy: A new approach. *Perspectives on Politics, 9*(2), 247–267.

Corbett, J., & Veenendaal, W. (2018). *Democracy in small states: Persisting against all odds.* Oxford University Press.

Cornwell, A. (2021, January 16). Expo organisers prepare to hold Dubai event delayed by coronavirus. REUTERS. Retrieved from: https://www.reuters.com/article/us-dubai-expo-idUSKBN29L0I4. Accessed 24 Oct 2021.

Corpuz, J. C. G. (2021). Adapting to the culture of 'new normal': An emerging response to COVID-19. *Journal of Public Health, 43*(2), e344–e345. https://doi.org/10.1093/pubmed/fdab057

Cotula, L. (2021). Towards a political economy of the COVID-19 crisis: Reflections on an agenda for research and action. *World Development, 138*, 105235.

Cotula, L., & Schwartz, B. (2020). COVID-19 and global economic ordering: Radical shift or more of the same? *International Institute for Environment and Development.* Retrieved from: https://www.iied.org/covid-19-global-economic-ordering-radical-shift-or-more-same

Cox, J. (2021, October 12). A record 4.3 million workers quit their jobs in August, led by food and retail industries. *CNBC.* Retrieved from: https://www.cnbc.com/2021/10/12/a-record-4po int3-million-workers-quit-their-jobs-in-august-led-by-food-and-retail-industries.html. Accessed 13 Nov 2021.

Crawley, H. (2019). Why equality matters if we want to harness the benefits of migration. *MIDEQ Blog.* Retrieved from: https://www.mideq.org/en/blog/why-equality-matters-if-we-want-harness-benefits-migration/. Accessed 4 Aug 2021.

Crawley, H. (2020). The great amplifier: COVID-19, migration and inequality. *MIDEQ Blog.* Retrieved from: https://www.mideq.org/en/blog/great-amplifier-covid-19-migration-and-inequa lity/. Accessed 4 Aug 2021.

Dahl, R. A. (1971). *Polyarchy: Participation and opposition.* Yale University Press.

Dauba-Pantanacce, P. (2020, April 20). The political implications of COVID-19. *Standard Chartered.* Retrieved from: https://www.sc.com/en/feature/the-political-implications-of-covid-19/. Accessed 30 July 2021.

Donaghy, E., Atherton, H., Hammersley, V., McNeilly, H., Bikker, A., Robbins, L., Campbell, J., & McKinstry, B. (2019). Acceptability, benefits, and challenges of video consulting: A qualitative study in primary care. *British Journal of General Practice, 69*(686), e586–e594.

Downs, A. (1957). *An economic theory of democracy.* Harper.

Du, J., Delis, A., Douch, M., & Shepotylo, O. (2020). Coronavirus won't kill globalization—But a shakeup is inevitable. *The Conversation.* Retrieved from: https://theconversation.com/corona virus-wont-kill-globalisation-but-a-shakeup-is-inevitable-137847

Earnshaw, V. (2020). Don't let the fear of Covid-19 turn into Stigma. *Economics and Society.* Retrieved from: https://hbr.org/2020/04/dont-let-fear-of-covid-19-turn-into-stigma. Accessed 06 Aug 2020.

Eden, A., et al. (2001). Involvement of branched-chain amino acid aminotransferases in the production of fusel alcohols during fermentation in yeast. *Applied Microbiology and Biotechnology, 55*(3), 296–300.

Enderwick, P., & Buckley, P. J. (2020). Rising regionalization: Will the post-COVID-19 world see a retreat from globalization? *Transnational Corporations Journal, 27*(2), 99–112.

European Institute of Peace (EIP). (2020). *The impact of Covid-19 on conflict affected and fragile states*. Retrieved from: https://www.eip.org/the-impact-of-covid-19-on-conflict-affected-and-fra gile-states/. Accessed 15 Nov 2021.

Faiola, A. (2020). The virus that shutdown the world. *The Washington Post*. Retrieved from: https://www.washingtonpost.com/graphics/2020/world/coronavirus-pandemic-globaliza tion/. Accessed 5 May 2021.

Falleti, T. G., & Lynch, J. F. (2009). Context and causal mechanisms in political analysis. *Comparative Political Studies, 42*(9), 1143–1166. https://doi.org/10.1177/0010414009331724

Fannin, R. (2020, March 2). The rush to deploy robots in China amid the coronavirus outbreak. *CNBC*. Retrieved from: https://www.cnbc.com/2020/03/02/the-rush-to-deploy-robots-in-china-amid-the-coronavirus-outbreak.html. Accessed 3 May 2021.

Fauvelle-Aymar, C., & François, A. (2018). Place of registration and place of residence: The non-linear detrimental impact of transportation cost on electoral participation. *Public Choice, 176*(3), 405–440.

Fernando, R., & McKibbin, W. J. (2021). Macroeconomic policy adjustments due to COVID-19: Scenarios to 2025 with a focus on Asia. In B. John, P. J. Morgan, & T. Sonobe (Eds.), *COVID-19 impacts and policy options: An Asian perspective* (pp. 399–472). Asian Development Bank.

Fontaine, R. (2020, April 17). Globalization will look very different after the coronavirus pandemic. *Foreign Policy*. Retrieved from: https://foreignpolicy.com/2020/04/17/globalization-trade-war-after-coronavirus-pandemic/. Accessed 17 May 2021.

Fujiwara, T. (2015). Voting technology, political responsiveness, and infant health: Evidence from Brazil. *Econometrica, 83*(2), 423–464.

Garattini, C., Raffle, J., Aisyah, D. N., Sartain, F., & Kozlakidis, Z. (2019). Big data analytics, infectious diseases and associated ethical impacts. *Philosophy & Technology, 32*(1), 69–85.

Gilmore, B., Ndejjo, R., Tchetchia, A., de Claro, V., Mago, E., Diallo, A. A., Lopes, C., & Bhat-tacharyya, S. (2020). Community engagement for COVID-19 prevention and control: A rapid evidence synthesis. BMJ Glob Health. 5(10):e003188. https://www.ncbi.nlm.nih.gov/pubmed/33051285

Goetz, K. H., & Martinsen, D. S. (2021). COVID-19: A dual challenge to European liberal democracy. *West European Politics, 44*(5–6), 1003–1024. https://doi.org/10.1080/01402382.2021.193 0463

Gomez, B. T., Hansford, T. G., & Krause, G. A. (2007). The Republicans should pray for rain: Weather, turnout, and voting in US presidential elections. *The Journal of Politics, 69*(3), 649–663.

Gordon, D. F. (2020). The coronavirus pandemic and global politics: Impact on major trends in security, health and governance, and great-power politics. *The International Institute for Strategic Studies*. Retrieved from: https://www.iiss.org/blogs/research-paper/2020/12/strategic-geo-economic-implications-covid-19-pandemic. Accessed 30 July 2021.

Guillen, M. (2020). The Politics of pandemic. *Strategic Policy, Strategic Survey, 120*(1), 25–78. https://doi.org/10.1080/04597230.2020.1835086

Hatuel-Radoshitzkey, M., & Heistein, A. (2020). Global governance and COVID-19: Why international cooperation still matters. In T. Bernes, L. Brozus, M. Hatuel-radoshitzky, A. Heistein, E. Greco et al. (Eds.), *Challenges of global governance amid the COVID-19 pandemic*. Council on Foreign Relations.

Hick, J. L., Hanfling, D., Wynia, M. K., & Pavia, A. T. (2020). *Duty to plan: Health care, crisis standards of care, and novel coronavirus SARS-CoV-2. Nam Perspectives*. National Academy of Medicine.

Human Rights Watch. (2020, March 19). *Human rights dimensions of COVID-19 response*. Retrieved from: https://www.hrw.org/news/2020/03/19/human-rights-dimensions-covid-19-res ponse#_Toc35446577. Accessed 13 July 2021.

Human Rights Watch. (2021a). *Covid-19 triggers wave of free speech abuse*. Retrieved from: https://www.hrw.org/news/2021/02/11/covid-19-triggers-wave-free-speech-abuse. Accessed 18 July 2021.

References

Human Rights Watch. (2021b). *Pandemic's dire global impact on education.* Retrieved from: https://www.hrw.org/news/2021/05/17/pandemics-dire-global-impact-education. Accessed 16 July 2021.

Igoye, A. (2020). Migration and immigration: Uganda and the COVID-19 pandemic. *Public Integrity, 22*(4), 406–408. https://doi.org/10.1080/10999922.2020.1753383

International Institute for Democracy and Electoral Assistance (IDEA). (2021). *Global overview of COVID-19: Impact on elections.* Retrieved from: https://www.idea.int/news-media/multimedia-reports/global-overview-covid-19-impact-elections. Accessed 9 July 2021.

International Labor Organization (ILO). (2011). Social protection floor for a fair and inclusive globalization: Report of the Advisory Group chaired by Michelle Bachelet Convened by the ILO with the collaboration of the WHO. International Labor Organization. Retrieved from: https://www.ilo.org/wcmsp5/groups/public/---dgreports/---dcomm/---publ/doc uments/publication/wcms_165750.pdf. Accessed 20 Sept 2020.

International Labour Organization (ILO). (2020a, June 19). *Reaching women migrant workers in Malaysia amid the COVID 19 health crisis.* Retrieved from: https://www.ilo.org/asia/media-cen tre/articles/WCMS_751495/lang--en/index.htm

International Labour Organization (ILO). (2020b). COVID-19: *Impact on migrant workers and country response in Thailand.* Retrieved from: https://www.ilo.org/wcmsp5/groups/public/---asia/---ro-bangkok/---sro-bangkok/documents/briefingnote/wcms_741920.pdf. Accessed 30 July 2021.

International Labour Organization (ILO). (2020c). *The COVID 19 response: Getting gender equality right for a better future for women at work.* Available at https://www.ilo.org/wcmsp5/groups/pub lic/---dgreports/---gender/documents/publication/wcms_744685.pdf. Accessed 30 July 2021.

International Labour Organization (ILO). (2020d). *COVID-19 and the world of work* (1st ed.).

International Labour Organization (ILO). (2020e). A policy framework for tackling the economic and social impact of the COVID-19 crisis. *ILO Brief.* Retrieved from: https://www.ilo.org/wcm sp5/groups/public/@dgreports/@dcomm/documents/briefingnote/wcms_745337.pdf. Accessed 06 July 2021.

International Organization for Migration (IOM). (2021). *IOM Strategic Response and Recovery Plan COVID-19.* International Organization for Migration.

Josephson, J., Wolfgang, C., & Mehrenberg, R. (2018). Strategies for supporting students who are twice-exceptional. *The Journal of Special Education Apprenticeship, 7*(2), Article 8. Available at: https://scholarworks.lib.csusb.edu/josea/vol7/iss2/8

Kalpana, P., Patel, K., Yasobant, S., & Saxena, D. B. (2021). Water, Sanitation, and Hygiene (WASH) during COVID19 pandemic in India: Practicability in poor settings! *Social Sciences & Humanities Open, 4*(1), 100195. https://www.ncbi.nlm.nih.gov/pubmed/34308337

Kandel, N., Chungong, S., Omaar, A., & Xing, J. (2020). Health security capacities in the context of COVID-19 outbreak: An analysis of International Health Regulations annual report data from 182 countries. *The Lancet, 395*(10229), 1047–1053.

Kaur, R. J., Dutta, S., Bhardwaj, P., Charan, J., Dhingra, S., Mitra, P., Singh, K., Yadav, D., Sharma, P., & Misra, S. (2021). Adverse events reported from COVID-19 vaccine trials: A systematic review. *Indian Journal of Clinical Biochemistry,* 1–13. https://www.ncbi.nlm.nih.gov/pubmed/33814753

Kelly, J. (2020). *Here are the big winners and losers in our new post-Covid-19 world.* Retrieved from: https://www.forbes.com/sites/jackkelly/2020/05/18/here-are-the-big-winners-and-losers-in-our-new-post-covid-19-world/?sh=1d34484fd2c0. Accessed 20 July 2021.

Klein, N., Smith, N., & Patrick, C. (2008). The shock doctrine: A discussion. *Environment and Planning d: Society and Space, 26*(4), 582–595.

Kolie, D., Delamou, A., van de Pas, R., Dioubate, N., Bouedouno, P., Beavogui, A. H., Diallo, A. M., Van De Put, W., & Van Damme, W. (2019). 'Never let a crisis go to waste': Post-Ebola agenda-setting for health system strengthening in Guinea. *BMJ Global Health, 4*(6), e001925.

Lee, G. (2020, July 21). Coronavirus: EU leaders reach recovery deal after marathon summit. *BBC News, 21.* Retrieved from: https://www.bbc.com/news/world-europe-53481542

Lindberg, S. I. (2013). Mapping accountability: Core concept and subtypes. *International Review of Administrative Sciences, 79*(2), 202–226.

Logie, C. H., & Turan, J. M. (2020). How do we balance tensions between COVID-19 public health responses and stigma mitigation? Learning from HIV research. *AIDS and Behavior, 24*(7), 2003–2006.

Ma, R., Zheng, X., Wang, P., Liu, H., & Zhang, C. (2021). The prediction and analysis of COVID-19 epidemic trend by combining LSTM and Markov method. *Scientific Reports, 11*(1), 1–14.

Mahoney, J. (2001). Leadership skills for the 21st century. *Journal of Nursing Management, 9*(5), 269–271. https://doi.org/10.1046/j.1365-2834.2001.00230.x

Mattiuzzi, C., & Lippi, G. (2020). Which lessons shall we learn from the 2019 novel coronavirus outbreak? *Annals of Translational Medicine, 8*(3), 48.

McKibbin, W., & Vines, D. (2020). Global macroeconomic cooperation in response to the COVID-19 pandemic: A roadmap for the G20 and the IMF. *Oxford Review of Economic Policy, 36*(1), 297–337.

Mega, E. R. (2020). Latin America's embrace of an unproven COVID treatment is hindering drug trials. *Nature, 586*(7830), 481–483.

Merkel, W. (2004). Embedded and defective democracies. *Democratization, 11*(5), 33–58.

Miller, O. (2021, January 15). *Covid-19 has taught us how to prepare for future pandemics.* Retrieved from https://www.kent.ac.uk/news/science/27658/expert-comment-covid-19-has-already-taught-us-how-to-prepare-for-future-pandemics. Accessed 13 May 2021.

Mohan, D. (2020a). *A broad crisis of public distrust that we need to resolve.* Retrieved from: http://dspace.jgu.edu.in:8080/jspui/bitstream/10739/4281/1/A%20broad%20crisis%20of%20public%20distrust%20.pdf. Accessed 30 July 2021.

Mohan, D. (2020b, May 2). The geopolitical contours of a post-COVID-19 world. *East Asia Forum.* Retrieved from: https://www.eastasiaforum.org/2020/05/02/the-geopolitical-contours-of-a-post-covid-19-world/. Accessed 30 July 2021.

Mueller, D. C. (2003). *Public choice III.* Cambridge University Press.

Muggah, R., & Katz, R. (2020, March 17). How cities around the world are handling COVID-19-and why we need to measure their preparedness. *World Economic Forum.* Retrieved from: https://smartnet.niua.org/sites/default/files/resources/covid-19_how_cities_around_the_world_are_coping_world_economic_forum.pdf. Accessed 29 July 2021.

Neate, R. (2020, October 7). Billionaires' wealth rises to $10.2 trillion amid Covid crisis. *The Guardian.* Retrieved from: https://www.theguardian.com/business/2020/oct/07/covid-19-crisis-boosts-the-fortunes-of-worlds-billionaires. Accessed 1 Aug 2021.

O'Meara, S. (2020). Meet the engineer behind China's first robot-run coronavirus ward. *Nature, 582*(7813), S53–S53.

OECD. (2019). *Social spending.* Retrieved from: https://data.oecd.org/socialexp/social-spending.htm. Accessed 8 Mar 2021.

OECD. (2020a, November 10). The territorial impact of COVID-19: Managing the crisis across levels of government. *OECD.* Retrieved from: https://www.oecd.org/coronavirus/policy-responses/the-territorial-impact-of-covid-19-managing-the-crisis-across-levels-of-government-d3e314e1/. Accessed 9 Mar 2021.

OECD. (2020b). Unemployment Rates, OECD—Updated: November 2020b. Retrieved from: http://www.oecd.org/sdd/labour-stats/unemployment-rates-oecd-update-november-2020.htm. Accessed 12 Oct 2021.

Osman, M. E. (2020). Global impact of COVID-19 on education systems: The emergency remote teaching at Sultan Qaboos University. *Journal of Education for Teaching, 46*(4), 463–471.

Panda, S., Kaur, H., Dandona, L., & Bhargava, B. (2021). Face mask—An essential armour in the fight of India against COVID-19. *Indian Journal of Medical Research, 153*(1 & 2), 233–237. https://www.ncbi.nlm.nih.gov/pubmed/33533732

Pariès, J. (2020). *What does the Covid-19 crisis teach us about resilience?* Institute for an Industrial Safety Culture, Retrieved from: https://www.icsi-eu.org/en/publication/tribuna-resilience-Covid-19. Accessed 11 Feb 2021.

References

149

Parker, K., Minkin, R., & Bennett, J. (2020). *Economic fallout from COVID-19 continues to hit lower-income Americans the hardest* (p. 21). Pew Research Center.

Pearson, J. (2020, December 3). Why COVID-19 shows the future not the end of globalization. *World Economic Forum.* Retrieved from: https://www.weforum.org/agenda/2020/12/covid-19-future-of-globalization-trade/. Accessed 6 Feb 2021.

Posel, D., Oyenubi, A., & Kollamparambil, U. (2021). Job loss and mental health during the COVID-19 lockdown: Evidence from South Africa. *PloS One, 16*(3), e0249352.

Quarantelli, E. L., & Dynes, R. R. (1977). Response to social crisis and disaster. *Annual Review of Sociology, 3,* 23–49. https://doi.org/10.1146/annurev.so.03.080177.000323

Rahmadhani, P., Vaz, F., & Affiat, R. A. (2021). *COVID-19 Crisis and women in Asia: Economic impacts and policy responses.* Friedrich-Ebert-Stiftung.

Ravi, S. J., Snyder, M. R., & Rivers, C. (2019). Review of international efforts to strengthen the global outbreak response system since the 2014–16 West Africa Ebola Epidemic. *Health Policy and Planning, 34*(1), 47–54.

Reddy KS. (2021). Pandemic lessons from India. *BMJ.* 373, n1196. https://www.ncbi.nlm.nih.gov/pubmed/33980588

Richter, F. (2021). COVID-19 has caused a huge amount of lost working hours. *World Economic Forum.* Retrieved from: https://www.weforum.org/agenda/2021/02/covid-employment-global-job-loss/. Accessed 18 Feb 2021.

Riker, W. H., & Ordeshook, P. C. (1968). A theory of the calculus of voting. *American Political Science Review, 62*(1), 25–42.

Rippert, A. (2021, June 10). What globalization will look like after COVID. *Fortune.* Retrieved from: https://fortune.com/2021/06/10/globalization-after-covid-tech-ai-netflix-accenture-edge-organizations/. Accessed 19 Feb 2021.

Rodriguez-Morales, A. J., Cardona-Ospina, J. A., & Gutiérrez-Ocampo, E. (2020). Going global—Travel and the 2019 novel coronavirus. *Travel Medicine and Infectious Disease, 33,* 101578. https://doi.org/10.1016/j.tmaid.2020.101578

Rosenthal, U., Charles, M. T., & 't Hart, P. (Eds.) (1989). *Coping with crises: The management of disasters, riots and terrorism.* Charles C. Thomas Publishers.

Rust, l. (2020). *Colorado issues guidance on accommodations in the age of COVID-19.* https://www.jdsupra.com/authors/laurie-rust/coronavirus-covid-19/

Saran, S. (2020, November 25). The Covid-19 pandemic and the shift in domestic politics. *The Hindustan Times.* Retrieved from: https://www.hindustantimes.com/india-news/htls-2020-the-covid-19-pandemic-and-the-shift-in-domestic-politics/story-zr65elSbG28964MMznFbRP.html. Accessed 15 Oct 2021.

Sawada, Y., & Sumulong, L. R. (2021). Macroeconomic impacts of the COVID-19 pandemic in developing Asia. In J. Beirne, P. J. Morgan, & T. Sonobe (Eds), *COVID-19 impacts and policy options: An Asian perspective* (pp. 11–47). Asian Development Bank.

Schedler, A. (1999). Conceptualizing accountability. In A. Schedler, L. J. Diamond, & M. F. Plattner, (Eds.). (1999). *The self-restraining state: Power and accountability in New Democracies* (pp. 13–28). Lynne Rienner.

Sharma, I., Vashnav, M., & Sharma, R. (2020). COVID-19 pandemic hype: Losers and gainers. *Indian Journal of Psychiatry, 62*(Suppl 3), S420. Retrieved from: https://doi.org/10.4103/psychiatry.IndianJPsychiatry_1060_20

Shinozaki, S., & Rao, L. N. (2021). Impacts of COVID-19 on micro, small, and medium-sized enterprises under lockdown: Evidence from a rapid survey in the Philippines. In J. Beirne, P. J. Morgan, & T. Sonobe (Eds.), *COVID-19 impacts and policy options: An Asian perspective* (pp. 140–187). Asian Development Bank.

Slipowitz, A. (2021, September 27). The devastating impact of COVID-19 on democracy. *Think Global Health.* Retrieved from: https://www.thinkglobalhealth.org/article/devastating-impact-covid-19-democracy. Accessed 13 Dec 2021.

Smith, J. F. (2021, March 31). Fallacies, hard truths, and lessons learned from the global response to COVID-19. *Harvard Kennedy School.* Retrieved from: https://www.hks.harvard.edu/faculty-res

earch/policy-topics/health/fallacies-hard-truths-and-lessons-learned-global-response. Accessed 30 July 2021.

Sonobe, T., Asami, T., Yoshida, S., & Truong, H. T. (2021). COVID-19 Impacts on micro, small, and medium-sized enterprises in Asia and their digitalization responses. In J. Beirne, P. J. Morgan, & T. Sonobe (Eds.), *COVID-19 impacts and policy options: An asian perspective* (pp. 96–139). Asian Development Bank.

Šumonja, M. (2020). Neoliberalism is not dead—On political implications of Covid-19. *Capital & Class*, 0309816820982381. Retrieved from: https://doi.org/10.1177/0309816820982381

Thakur, R. (2020, June 5). Coronavirus winners and losers. *Australian Strategic Policy Institute*. Retrieved from: https://www.aspistrategist.org.au/coronavirus-winners-and-losers/. Accessed 26 Aug 2021.

Thangavel, P., Pathak, P., & Chandra, B. (2021). Covid-19: Globalization—Will the course change? *Vision*. Retrieved from: https://doi.org/10.1177/0972262920984571

Tsoukalis, L. (2012). The political economy of the crisis: The end of an era? *Global Policy, 3*(1), 42–50.

Ullah, A. A. (2016). *Globalization and the health of Indigenous peoples: From colonization to self-rule*. Routledge.

Ullah, A. A., & Ming Yit Ho, H. (2021). Globalisation and cultures in Southeast Asia: Demise, fragmentation, transformation. *Global Society, 35*(2), 191–206.

Ullah, A. A., Hasan, N. H., Mohamad, S. M., & Chattoraj, D. (2020). Migration and security: Implications for minority migrant groups. *India Quarterly, 76*(1), 136–153.

Ullah, A. A., Hasan, N. H., Mohamad, S. M., & Chattoraj, D. (2021). Privileged migrants and their sense of belonging: Insider or outsider? *Asian Journal of Social Science, 49*(3), 161–169.

Ullah, A. A., Hossain, M. A., & Chattoraj, D. (2020). Covid-19 and Rohingya refugee camps in Bangladesh. *Intellectual Discourse, 28*(2), 793–806.

Ullah, A. A., Hossain, M. A., & Huque, A. S. (2021). Non-conventional migration: An evolving pattern in South Asia. *Journal of African and Asian Studies, 56*(3), 00219096211008468.

Ullah, A. A., Kumpoh, A. A. Z. A., & Haji-Othman, N. A. (2021). Covid-19 vaccine and international relations: New frontiers of vaccine diplomacy. *Southeast Asia: A Multidisciplinary Journal, 21*(1), 1–14.

Ullah, A. A., Lee, S. C. W., Hassan, N. H., & Nawaz, F. (2020). Xenophobia in the GCC countries: Migrants' desire and distress. *Global Affairs, 6*(2), 203–223.

Ullah, A. A., Nawaz, F., & Chattoraj, D. (2021). Locked up under lockdown: The COVID-19 pandemic and the migrant population. *Social Sciences & Humanities Open, 3*(1), 1–5. Retrieved from: https://doi.org/10.1016/j.ssaho.2021.100126

Ullah, A. K. M., Hossain, M. A., Azizuddin, M., & Nawaz, F. (2020). Social research methods: Migration in perspective. *Migration Letters, 17*(2), 357–368.

Ullah, A. K. M. A., Haji-Othman, N. A., & Daud, M. K. (2021). COVID-19 and shifting border policies in Southeast Asia. *Southeast Asia: A Multidisciplinary Journal, 21*(2), 1–14.

UNAIDS. (2020). Addressing stigma and discrimination in the COVID-19 response. Retrieved from https://www.unaids.org/sites/default/files/media_asset/covid19-stigma-brief_en.pdf. Accessed 5 Aug 2021.

UNESCO. (2020). *Education: From disruption to recovery*. https://en.unesco.org/covid19/educationresponse

UNICEF. (2020). Education and COVID-19. Retrieved from: https://data.unicef.org/topic/education/covid-19/. Accessed 9 Aug 2021.

United Nations (UN). (2020). Policy brief: Education during COVID-19 and beyond, August 2020. Retrieved from: https://www.un.org/development/desa/dspd/wp-content/uploads/sites/22/2020/08/sg_policy_brief_covid-19_and_education_august_2020.pdf. Accessed 14 Aug 2021.

Ward, P. R. (2020). A sociology of the Covid-19 pandemic: A commentary and research agenda for sociologists. *Journal of Sociology, 56*(4), 726–735.

References

Wintour, P. (2020, April 11). Coronavirus: Who will be winners and losers in new world order? *The Guardian*. Retrieved from: https://www.theguardian.com/world/2020/apr/11/coronavirus-who-will-be-winners-and-losers-in-new-world-order. Accessed 1 Sept 2021.

Woods, E. T., Schertzer, R., Greenfeld, L., Hughes, C., & Miller-Idriss, C. (2020). COVID-19, nationalism, and the politics of crisis: A scholarly exchange. *Nations and Nationalism, 26*(4), 807–825.

Worldometers. (2021). *Coronavirus updates*. https://www.worldometers.info/coronavirus/

Yaakop, M. R., Ali, S. A. A. D. S., Taib, R., Mohamad, A. R., & Razif, M. A. M. (2020). Malaysia Political Changes amid Covid-19. *International Journal of Academic Research in Business and Social Sciences, 10*(12), 224–233.

Youngs, R., & Panchulidze, E. (2020). Global democracy & Covid-19: Upgrading international support. *European Endowment for Democracy*. Retrieved from: https://www.democracyendowment.eu/en/news/1741-global-democracy-and-covid-19-upgrading-international-support.html. Accessed 19 July 2021.

Yurgens, I. (2020). *COVID-19 and rebalancing the global agenda. Challenges of global governance amid the COVID-19 pandemic*. Council on Foreign Relations: International Institutions and Global Governance Program.

Zhong, L. (2021). A dynamic pandemic model evaluating reopening strategies amid COVID-19. *PloS one, 16*(3), e0248302.

Zhou, X., Snoswell, C. L., Harding, L. E., Bambling, M., Edirippulige, S., Bai, X., & Smith, A. C. (2020, Apr). The role of telehealth in reducing the mental health burden from COVID-19. *Telemedicine and e-Health, 26*(4), 377–379. https://doi.org/10.1089/tmj.2020.0068. Epub 2020 Mar 23. PMID: 32202977.

Zwitter, A. (2012). The Rule of law in times of crisis a legal theory on the state of emergency in the liberal democracy. *Archiv Für Rechts-Und Sozialphilosphie, 98*(1), 95–111.

Chapter 5
Choosing to End the Pandemic: Conclusions and Discussion

Introduction

Due to the second-quarter transition to normalcy, a number of countries like the United States, Canada, and Western Europe have enjoyed some relief from the COVID-19 epidemic since March 2021. The high-income countries' expectations of a return to normalcy were hindered by cases caused by the Delta strain. After a delayed start, Western Europe and Canada will overtake the United States in the first quarter of 2021 in terms of the number of completely immunized citizens (Flanagan, 2021). According to scientists, this progress has been enabled by rapid vaccine distribution. Yet, due to the emergence of the more transmissible and lethal Delta and Omicron variants and the continuance of hesitancy about the vaccine, that share has been insufficient to achieve herd immunity (Vogel & Eggertson, 2020). In the short term, the Delta variant raises the disease burden by increasing the number of cases, hospitalizations, and deaths, and Delta's high transmissibility also makes obtaining herd immunity more difficult (World Economic Forum, 2021).

As COVID-19 swept around the world in 2020, affluent countries spent billions of dollars accelerating vaccine development and procuring early supplies. A vigorous advertising effort is employed to allay customers' concerns about the quality of any new product entering the market. Over seven immunizations have shown promise in the fight against COVID-19. These are brand-new products developed and purchased by various governments throughout the world for marketing purposes. As is the case with many other vaccines on the market, these vaccines are composed of a variety of components and concentrations (Mogaji, 2021). If governments are trying to protect their citizens from this epidemic that has killed nearly 5 million people, damaged economies, and wreaked devastation around the world how much should pharmaceutical firms charge?

By 2021, it is estimated that the market for COVID vaccines will exceed $100 billion. While both Pfizer and Moderna announced combined vaccine sales of $17.2 billion in the first half of 2021, both firms are anticipated to make total vaccine sales of $18 billion in late November 2021. In the first half of 2021, Pfizer made $11.3

© The Author(s), under exclusive license to Springer Nature Singapore Pte Ltd. 2022 153
AKM. A. Ullah and J. Ferdous, *The Post-Pandemic World and Global Politics*,
https://doi.org/10.1007/978-981-19-1910-7_5

billion in revenue from its COVID-19 vaccine, which is now known as Comirnaty. Analysts predict that Pfizer will make $11.86 billion in revenue in the third quarter. Those projections, however, may be exaggerated because some sales may be pushed into the fourth quarter, when booster doses and the newly permitted vaccination for younger children begin to arrive.

The most anticipated beneficiaries are Moderna Inc. and Pfizer Inc., as well as China's Sinovac Biotech Ltd. and Sinopharm Group Co. According to sources from London School of Economics and Political Science and other universities, at least $10 billion has been invested in vaccines by Moderna, Johnson & Johnson, AstraZeneca Plc, and Pfizer's German partner BioNTech SE, among others. Public investment in COVID vaccinations has topped $50 billion, according to the Graduate Institute of International and Development Studies' (GIIDS) Global Health Centre in Geneva.

While vaccines used in Western countries remain very effective in preventing serious diseases caused by COVID-19, new research findings from Israel, the United Kingdom, and the United States cast doubt on the ability to prevent infection with the Delta and Omicron variants (Flanagan, 2021). This has prompted a number of countries to begin delivering booster doses to at-risk individuals or to plan for their use (World Economic Forum, 2021).

The COVID-19 pandemic is the subject of scenarios like this one. Despite their differing timetables and projections, forecasters agree on the following two points: No one knows how long people will be able to resist COVID-19, if seasonality has any effect on its spread, and—perhaps most importantly—the decisions governments and individuals will make in the next years (Scudellari, 2020). This has raised new concerns about the fact that when the world can expect the pandemic to end. However, the example of the UK suggests that if a country has weathered a Delta-driven surge of cases, it may be able to relax public health restrictions and return to normalcy. Beyond that, a more realistic epidemiological goal may be attained when countries can handle COVID-19 as an endemic infection rather than when herd immunity is acquired (Ullah et al., 2021). The emergence of a new variant that is more transmissible, more likely to result in hospitalizations and fatalities, or more capable of infecting individuals who have been vaccinated would thus likely pose the biggest threat to a country's ability to do so (World Economic Forum, 2021).

There is no doubt that raising immunization rates is crucial for restoring normalcy. On the other hand, vaccine reluctance has proven to be a persistent impediment to preventing the spread of the Delta strain. Vaccines have been made available to adolescents and children soon, protecting a demographic segment that makes for a large share of the population in various countries (World Economic Forum, 2021). Vaccine politics have made it notoriously difficult to distribute vaccines and get individuals immunized in emerging and undeveloped countries. Some media entities have been seen to come forward in order to spark political debate about the pandemic. For example, some media outlets in South Asia (especially in India) and North America are adamant that the virus's name be changed to the Wuhan virus, while the Indian variant has been termed delta variant. A pandemic is a pandemic that should be fought together without undermining any country in any way. Hence,

Introduction   155

the WHO Director-General said, the pandemic will come to an end when the world decides to end it (WHO, 2021).

The first chapter introduces the book and elaborates on the research on which the book is based. The chapter is divided into three sections: the literature review, arguments, the study methodology, and the data analysis. The chapter emphasizes the relevance of the book and how it is designed to provide an overview of the subject matter. We attempt to depict how global politics has evolved and how the politicization of the COVID-19 outbreak affects global health inequities.

The second chapter addresses the magnitude of the pandemic as well as some conceptual concerns that explain the current situation. According to proponents of globalization theory, the world has devolved into "one-world," or a single global community. This indicates that the entire globe had grown into a global society. The implication is that something that happens in one region of the world swiftly spreads to the rest of the world. As global problems, crises, and difficulties arose, necessitating international collaboration and nations working together in a culture of "complex interdependence," international relations were elevated to the level of global politics.

The third chapter goes into politics, its outcomes, and its consequences. COVID-19 is a shock to the global order, changing global politics and sparking new wars between friends and rivals. It will have long-term geopolitical consequences. Difficulties have plagued international politics. The gap between public and private goods was growing, and multilateralism was being questioned. The COVID-19 pandemic, on the other hand, has expedited these changes while also providing a new chance to reproduce the global politics, economy and security.

The fourth chapter discusses predictions for the post-COVID world and politics and what the world should and could do. The multiple implications of COVID-19 for individuals, groups, and regions, as well as the possibility of exacerbated territorial imbalances, need a place-based approach to regional development, more inclusivity, and a renewed sense of urgency. The importance of top-down and bottom-up activity balance, the necessity for successful connections and trust across several sets of actors, and the requirement for adaptability and flexibility contribute to this sense of urgency. Some interesting facts are laid out in the last chapter, and we attempt to come up with the path to solutions. In this chapter, we focus on the most important concepts that underlie the book's fundamental concerns. As a result of this pandemic, we discuss what we've learned and how global politics should evolve in the future.

Is everything Going to Change?

We believe the world will restructure politics and reshape public health investment programmes when this period is over. Even so, the collective spirit endures. The rest of the world will be able to see how our fortunes are interwoven. The cheap burger we buy from a business that refuses to provide paid sick leave to its employees, as well as our neighbour, who refuses to stay home during the pandemic because our public school failed to teach us critical thinking skills, make us more susceptible to the infection. Suppose the government does not provide income guarantees to the millions of employees who would lose their jobs. In that case, the economy will implode and the social order it serves to sustain. All religions have struggled to keep their faith in the face of adversity—but never all religions at the same time. During a quarantine period, religion puts conventional notions about what it means to comfort to the test. Individuals who do not belong to a local congregation, on the other hand, will be able to hear sermons from a distance. Contemplative activities have the potential to grow in popularity.

The enormous shock(s) that the coronavirus pandemic is bringing to our system can liberate us from the world's rising political and cultural polarization and assist us in reorienting ourselves toward greater national togetherness and functionality. While this may look idealistic, there are two reasons why we believe it is doable. The first scenario is the "shared adversary," in which people overcome their differences in response to a common external threat. COVID-19 is a formidable foe that will not distinguish between reds and blues and may provide us with fusion-like energy and a singularity of purpose to help us reset (Politico, 2020). The COVID-19 pandemic has driven individuals to see the value of knowledge. For example, everyone wanted to hear from doctors as the pandemic came. Second, it has the potential to reawaken people's sense of seriousness. For example, the Trump administration's colossal failure to keep the Americans safe and to halt the economy's pandemic-driven implosion may jolt the public into wanting something other than emotional comfort from the government. We risk devolving into authoritarianism. Consider the fact that President Donald Trump's request to delay the November election and the possibility of a military deployment. Our relationship with market culture and hyper-individualism is shattered as a result of the pandemic. We are currently witnessing the catastrophic breakdown of market-based social organization paradigms, as self-seeking behaviour exacerbates the situation far more than it needed to be (Politico, 2020).

This pandemic has appeared as a boon for virtual reality. Because of virtual reality, we can enjoy the experiences we want even when we are secluded, quarantined, or alone. COVID-19 removes a slew of artificial impediments to more of our lives being shared online. Of course, not everything can be virtualized. However, in many aspects of our life, the adoption of genuinely effective internet tools has been blocked by prominent legacy players who routinely collaborate with overly cautious authorities (Politico, 2020).

Telemedicine is not a new phenomenon, nor is it limited to the United States. One need only go to the islands of southern Italy, where a successful telemedicine programme has improved healthcare delivery to rural areas while also offering high-quality care (Betancourt et al., 2020). The use of telemedicine is on the rise. Telemedicine has been a low-cost, high-convenience option for many years. Remote office visits may become more common as the pandemic overwhelms medical facilities. Additional containment benefits can be gained by conducting a video conference from your home, such as keeping you out of the public transit system and away from the waiting area for critically ill patients (Betancourt et al., 2020).

Coronavirus has exposed basic vulnerabilities in our healthcare system as millions of families have been forced to deal with this disaster without a safety net. Families are ill and children are absent from school, so they are forced to choose between their health, their families, and financial ruin (Wong, 2021). Furthermore, there is a lack of effective child care support, inconsistency in long-term care access, and a lack of paid family and medical leave, which results in missed work and lost wages. A new political movement is envisaged as a result of the coronavirus. Our communities will be able to see how well-connected and resourced the well-off have fared during this health emergency and how marginalized and destitute areas have been decimated (Sands, 2020). While it is possible to mobilize billion-dollar bailouts and infrastructure projects rapidly, only if the need is deemed urgent, we will also have seen how political action may be mobilized.

In terms of election and politics, despite numerous complaints, electronic voting will become more common. The prior concept of limiting voting to polling stations where people must congregate in close proximity for a lengthy amount of time will be one of the casualties of COVID-19 (Flinders, 2021; Ashord & Kroenig, 2020). Many countries are gradually abandoning this strategy. Mail-in ballots may eventually become the standard. Many countries have rescheduled presidential and local government elections. Many other countries will almost certainly follow suit. These elections, however, cannot be postponed indefinitely. Parties must have conventions and choose representatives. According to some assessments, the coronavirus may continue to pose a threat to individuals. This shows that most countries' election policies are laying the groundwork for an electoral disaster.

We can expect additional restrictions on mass consumption in the future. We hope the pandemic's consequences will convince society to accept limits on mass consumer culture as a reasonable price for future contagious illness protection. For decades, we have satisfied our voracious appetites by conquering an ever-expanding region of the world with our industrial operations, forcing wild species to pack into diminishing patches of habitat closer to us. That is how animal viruses, such as SARS-COV2, as well as hundreds of others, such as Ebola and Zika, have infected people and caused epidemics (Shang et al., 2021).

The world economy is beginning to recover from the economic devastation caused by the coronavirus epidemic, with growth of 5.6 percent predicted for 2021. However, not everyone is experiencing this recovery in the same way. Global poverty is rising, and previously decreasing patterns of inequality are being reversed, as the poorer countries face a more severe and long-lasting crises. This means that the poorest individuals on the earth will bear the brunt of the COVID-19 pandemic. In 2021, the average global income of the bottom 40 percent will be 6.7 percent lower than pre-pandemic predictions, while the top 40 percent would see a 2.8 percent decline (World Bank, 2021). The reason for this gap is that the poorest 40 percent have yet to begin recovering their income losses, while the wealthiest 40 percent have recovered more than 45 percent of their initial income losses. The bottom 40 percent's average income fell by 2.2 percent between 2019 and 2021, while the top 40 percent's average income fell by 0.5 percent (Sánchez-Páramo et al., 2021).

158   5 Choosing to End the Pandemic: Conclusions and Discussion

As a result, the picture in the kitchen is changing as well. As a result of COVID-19, there will be less time for socializing and more time spent in the kitchen (Klaus & Christine, 2021). As a result, Americans have spent more money on eating out than they have on grocery shopping and preparing their own meals. With restaurants closing and individuals becoming more isolated, many people will learn or relearn how to cook in the coming weeks. Maybe they rediscover their love of cooking, though I doubt it, or maybe delivery will win out (Freedman, 2019).

International flows of information, money, products, and services have grown significantly over the previous three decades. National economies are being dismantled and reconstructed as global networks, stressing trade-offs and highlighting governance issues in a globally connected society. Instead of producing a Ricardian theory of win–win (Stigler, 1952) situations and increased prosperity for all, this deeply intertwined interdependence has created new vulnerabilities and sources of authority and influence among nation-states, enterprises, non-state actors, and within local political systems (Kurz, 2017). We describe major aspects of the changing political landscape of a post-pandemic period. Those who feel the breakout is a significant change from the past rather than a continuation of ongoing great power warfare are being called into doubt. Instead, we argue that the epidemic exacerbates pre-existing trends and forces scholars to reconsider their perspectives on globalization research.

Economic interdependence alters the significance of problems, as well as people's ability to overcome political conflicts. Of course, in a multitude of circumstances, including inequality and climate change, COVID-19 is not the primary source of conflict. As a result, the global pandemic serves as an excellent lens to evaluate, comprehend, and engage with future globalization politics. This goal involves scholars incorporating more notions of power and identity into their global market analyses, as well as acknowledging how globalization has altered political authority (McNamara & Newman, 2020). We go over a number of significant policy areas where globalization has a revolutionary impact, emphasizing how COVID-19 has brought these concerns to the forefront even further.

Implications for Politics

Some of the battles against the new coronavirus are being waged on a variety of fronts, including medical experts, governments, and even governments themselves trying to be seen as credible and effective leaders in the world. It appears that most governments are struggling to deal with the pandemic and regain the confidence of the general public.

Despite Japan's economic and technological capabilities, Japan's failings are remarkable in handling this pandemic. Critiques say that the epidemiologists and the administration had poor preparation to combat the pandemic. According to the most recent OECD figures, disasters kill more than four times as many people in Japan than in any other OECD country. Due to its high population density and international trade, Japan has five of the top twenty most densely populated metropolitan regions in the OECD's 300-city metropolitan database (Bolleyer & Salát, 2021; Glosserman, 2020). Japanese scientific study and adoption of international principles" allowed Japan to uncover and assess a number of important dangers and their potential public health consequences (OECD, 2021). Even though the government was aware of the threats, little was done about it. Planning ahead is the only way to ensure success in the real world. As demonstrated by the 1995 Great Hanshin Earthquake, the 1995 sarin attack on Tokyo subways, and the 2011 Great East Japan earthquake, crisis preparation is essential in the face of national calamities (The Japan Times, 2020).

Disaster risk reduction (DRR) was a major focus of Japan's 2015 World Conference on Disaster Risk Reduction (WCDRR). Japan's [then] Prime Minister Shinzo Abe presided over a G7 summit on global health a year after the conference. The G7's Ise-Shima Global Health Vision was endorsed by the organization. Complex disasters, like the Great East Japan Earthquake, showed the flaws in the method when faced with pre-planned emergency scenarios. Japan's preparation level is not reaching its full potential due to a lack of quality assurance at the local level, limited collaboration between ministries and levels of government, and an insufficient number of real-world exercises (Sakamoto et al., 2018). The widespread perception of Tokyo's capabilities is that the city handled the COVID-19 issue poorly. Regardless of Japan's technology and planning capabilities, the country's tale would be defined by its resilience, predilection for order, and capacity to work collaboratively toward a common goal. These national characteristics were abundantly seen before, during, and after Japan's 2011 "triple calamity" of earthquake, tsunami, and nuclear disaster. These characteristics can be used to galvanize the people and construct a more effective response to the disaster.

The most prevalent flu pandemics have originated in China. SARS (Severe Acute Respiratory Syndrome) killed 774 people in 17 countries; H7N9 (H7N9) killed over 1,200 people, killing 40% of them in 2012. During the current epidemic, Chinese cases increased substantially in the second half of 2021. Despite this, China's response to the pandemic has received widespread plaudits. There are reports, however, that after the WHO was notified of the coronavirus outbreak in China around the end of 2019, China was undermined by a political framework emphasizing the Chinese Communist Party's control over truth-telling because bad news was kept hidden since it was politically inconvenient. According to India, as concealment grew more difficult, the Chinese leadership changed the narrative from one of catastrophic failure to one of heroic measures to contain the virus. Both ensuring compliance and sending a strong message of leadership to the Chinese people were achieved by Beijing's extraordinary measures to combat swine flu, which included shutting down entire cities, making millions of people stay at home, and mobilizing the country's vast surveillance system to combat it all.

The WHO praised China's reaction, calling it the most daring, nimble, and aggressive disease management campaign. The West regards this as draconian. According to the WHO, "urgent access" to China's experience in responding to COVID-19 and the tangible commodities it gives to the global response are two items that must be made available as soon as possible. "China's amazing efforts in viral containment and commitment to global public health have earned China international esteem. A

160   5 Choosing to End the Pandemic: Conclusions and Discussion

country's reputation does not have to be defined by its first mistakes, as demonstrated by the Chinese example. But Tokyo must return to normalcy as quickly as possible (Ullah & Kumpoh, 2018, 2019; Glosserman, 2020).

Our greatest fear is that COVID-19 may spread to countries with less developed health systems, and the WHO pronouncement is not a vote of no confidence in China. In order to restrict and prevent the spread of COVID-19 across international borders, the international community needs to cooperate together (Dionne & Turkmen, 2020; Calisher et al., 2020). We need fast response times for active monitoring, early detection and isolation as well as contact tracking for these containment systems.

The unexpected halt in global mobility generated widespread worry among people, particularly migrant groups, many of whom were working in dangerous environments or were stranded at transit points where their dignity, security, and health were compromised (Ullah et al., 2019; Ullah et al. 2020c). As a result of border restrictions, asylum applicants were almost completely unable to get international protection. Despite some modest efforts to restore or transfer key infrastructure, foreign resettlement efforts have been considerably reduced as a result of stricter travel restrictions (Guadagno, 2020).

Thousands of migrants and travellers from all over the world have been imprisoned in countries with closed borders. Many people were forced to overstay their visas due to long-term travel restrictions in order to prevent the spread of the disease. When the restrictions were implemented, migrants on home leave or travelling outside of their host nation (even for visa renewal) were unable to return to their jobs, studies, homes, or families. Lockdowns and border restrictions caused a rapid return of migrants who had lost their social networks, professional chances and hope for a dignified life in their destination countries as a result of the epidemic. These occurrences jeopardize migrants' home countries and communities, as well as host and transit countries, in the global migratory network (Gunther, 2020; Joob & Wiwanitkit, 2020). Medical, childcare, and geriatric care, all of which rely heavily on immigration in industrialized economies, will see an increase in demand. As a result, migrant labour will likely be in higher demand (Dollar, 2020). Only citizens were permitted in due to lockdowns and emergency enacted in several countries. The government seemed to have a tendency to overlook the fact that many overseas couples are disqualified as they make polices of entries. They tend to forget that many residents married outside of the country. When countries only allow citizens, foreign husbands and wives are not permitted. This has resulted in a new type of separation experience for many people.

The epidemic will probably exacerbate the US's efforts to decouple China and encourage sectoral globalization. A new globality may emerge in some fields. The broader geopolitical ramifications—on the international system, inter-state competition, war, and coordination—are unlikely to yield a coherent overall picture: political will, negotiation, and international institutions' ability to participate (Rothgerber et al., 2020; Perthes, 2020). In light of the altering global landscape, both developed and developing countries can benefit from each other's expertise. The triangle alliance is recognized as an innovative technique for improving humanitarian aid efficacy. For the advantage of all three parties, a framework is established. Despite being

Implications for Politics

on a much smaller scale than North–South cooperation and having greater transaction costs, trilateral development cooperation has the potential to have a substantial impact on future international development collaboration. However, as a result of the epidemic, trilateral development cooperation has nearly come to a halt (Zhou et al., 2020).

The shift emphasizes a defining trait of modernity's future, namely continuous change, even while fundamental conceptions and underlying certainties remain constant. Metamorphosis, on the other hand, upends the fundamental pillars of modern civilisation. As a result, making predictions about the future is nearly impossible. However, we understand what must occur in order for mankind to emerge from this disaster in a better state than when it began. The idea that, in the absence of a revolution, the losers will always be the same: the poor, those refused aid, those with technological challenges, and migrants is a faulty but successful strategy. The most vulnerable will be recruited by the middle classes, who are now vulnerable yet want development through more comprehensive and accessible education. Certain advantages are made available by social insurance schemes and the steady growth of employment as a result of global trade. Assuming this is the case, governments all over the world should concentrate their efforts on preventing or, at the very least, reducing the repercussions. Financial aid to the world's poor, the concept of universal public healthcare for all individuals in a country or region, stricter regulations and natural resource preservation, and a focus on the underprivileged are just a few examples (Eiran, 2020).

COVID-19 risk is linked to human relationships, with persons with compromised immune systems or the elderly, as well as those who manifest readily, having a more significant probability of being impacted in congested urban regions with a higher population. Floating populations, slum dwellers, and individuals who rely on the city for a living have additional issues because they are more likely to lose jobs and money in the city. These people are highly vulnerable since they rely on daily income, have meagre or no savings, and are frequently enslaved by debt (GoB, 2020).

Aside from the costs of increasing poverty, interrupted lifestyles, lost vocations, and greater social unrest, the social costs of lost lives will have long-term consequences for global economic growth. By 2020, 95 million people are predicted to be living in poverty, an increase of 80 million from the pre-pandemic. Furthermore, other projections indicate that global trade will fall by 9.0 percent or less in 2020 as a result of the global economic crisis, wreaking havoc on trade-dependent emerging and developing economies in particular. In developed countries, the economic impact of the pandemic is projected to be mitigated because vaccines are expected to allow a recovery to pre-pandemic activity levels. On the other side, new virus strain infections in underdeveloped countries may extend the pandemic and make a recovery more challenging (CRS, 2021).

China began developing vaccinations in January 2020. Vaccines were developed through public–private partnerships that merged the resources of government research organizations with the manufacturing capabilities of pharmaceutical companies. Chinese vaccine companies conducted stage three research in developing countries all over the world, including Latin America, Africa, and the Middle East.

However, China had delays in exporting their vaccine. The KSA issued orders that those had Chinese vaccine would not be permitted to enter the country to perform Hajj. According to speculation, the under the dictation from the United States, the Saudi authorities issued this order.

While the primary purpose of clinical research funding in these states was to enhance vaccine access, China's "mask policy" aided this plan from the start. Vaccine developers frequently collaborated with the local pharmaceutical industry or public health agencies in exchange for a guaranteed price, delivery date, and technology transfer, which aided in participant recruitment, the establishment of physical and institutional resources, and the execution of studies. Assume a local pharmaceutical company paid for the clinical trial. In that instance, the agreement might declare that only in-country partners will be allowed to produce and distribute vaccines for local and global usage. Vaccines have been ordered in nearly every country where China conducted testing.

China considers vaccines to be "public goods" and has ensured that ASEAN and African countries have timely access to them and provide vaccine assistance to impoverished countries. For example, China delivered one million pills to Cambodia, 300,000 to Laos and Myanmar, and batches to Brunei and Nepal around Asia. China has sent dosages to a number of African countries, including the Democratic Republic of the Congo, Equatorial Guinea, and Sierra Leone. It has sent a small number of vaccines to Lebanon, Iraq, and Syria in the Middle East. On the other hand, these gifts are frequently offered and, in less quantities, than commercial contracts. It distributed 600,000 doses to the Philippines shortly after purchasing 25 million, 500,000 doses to Pakistan shortly after placing an order for 1.2 million doses, and 200,000 doses to Zimbabwe shortly after acquiring 600,000 doses (Yang, 2021). Almost half of the world's population has received COVID-19 vaccines. More than 7 billion immunizations have been administered. More than half of the world's countries, on the other hand, have barely inoculated a quarter of their citizens. Everyone does not receive the same number of vaccines: wealthier countries received roughly 50 times the number of Covid-19 vaccine doses as low-income countries. Low-income countries have the lowest rates of Covid-19 immunization. The majority of the population in many nations will not be protected against Covid-19 until well into 2022. Some of the world's poorest countries, for example, will not be there until 2023. There must be a reason for the slow pace. Hoarding is part of the story, but so are less-noticed hurdles including constrained supply chains and breakdowns in communication between vaccine makers, donors, and vaccination recipients (Irfan, 2021).

The existing system requires compliance with occupational health and safety rules, the provision of decent employment, and the preservation of labour rights across all industries. The first and most focused way to save lives and livelihoods should be to expand social welfare to include universal cure protection and economic assistance for the most disadvantaged. Among them are individuals in the informal economy and those in low-quality and low-paying employment, such as the elderly and migrants (Ullah, Hossain and Islam, 2015). To protect themselves and their families, women who work in low-wage jobs and are caretakers need to take extra precautions. Children's welfare payments and healthy school lunches, as well as

Implications for Politics 163

assistance with housing and food, employment retention/recovery, and financial aid for small businesses, are essential (WHO, 2020a).

During the COVID-19 outbreak, disputes between China, India, and the United States have reappeared. Is the current epidemic to blame for global hostility, or are these tensions the outcome of prior international cooperation? Is this a major issue that needs to be addressed? What are we doing in these challenging times when we should be uniting to save the world, and humanity? In reality, we are simply blaming one other for being to blame for the world's most critical problems. Unfortunately, human, the wisest race on the planet, has fallen to the COVID-19. At a minimum, the situation necessitates a global political solution rather than the formation of new crises. Will we be able to regain our composure and unite in the face of this pandemic? Finally, we would like to underline that the COVID-19's impact on global politics can be bad, as seen by current tensions between the US and China, and India and China.

COVID-19 has unfathomable political ramifications. Today's question is how seriously we take our commitments to the global brotherhood when we pledge mutual respect and support. Crises, such as the one we are currently experiencing expose the reality. Nations that should be cooperating accuse one another. We were unable to ascertain the dimensions that it has or will have an effect on. Rather than focusing just on the growth of a single nation, we should direct our efforts toward the greater good of humanity. We are humans, which is the most fundamental definition of who we are. National borders should not be used to determine our identities, particularly in the event of a pandemic. Of course, COVID-19 has a lot of global political implications, but it also has the potential to be a fantastic teacher for all of us, educating us about "the relevance and importance of all humanity's peaceful, safe, and harmonious lives."

According to numerous research, the COVID-19 pandemic had a significant influence on economic activity. Job loss or reduced hours, loss of sales and income from a home-based small business, inability to commute to work, increased time spent caring for children or sick family members, increased prices and/or lack of availability of necessities. Reduced access to education is all examples of the negative effects of the pandemic the world is going through. In times of reduced income, low-income people become more susceptible because they lack resources to draw from (Morgan & Trinh, 2021). People, governments and businesses are affected by pandemics by increasing business expenses, increasing public health care expenditures and modifying the labour supply due to mortality or disease. Consumption and production of perishable agricultural commodities, including meat and vegetables, have been severely affected (Morgan & Trinh, 2021; Nicola et al., 2020; Siche, 2020, Torero, 2020). Despite wide variations across countries, most households worldwide saw their income and employment drastically decrease.

Financial troubles were experienced by nearly half of all households. Around one-third of households in financial hardship were compelled to cut back on spending, while more than half depended on cash and savings. In order to get by, many borrowed monies from relatives and friends postponed payments and debt repayment, and/or applied for government assistance. In Morgan and Trinh's research (2021), nearly half of all households in their sample was able to manage for less than a month without any income at all. As a result, 27 percent of children were unable to return to school (particularly in Myanmar and the Philippines). Additionally, Morgan and Trinh (2021) found that male- and female-headed households were affected by the COVID-19 pandemic differently. For example, female-led households in the lower-income quartiles were more affected by income shocks than male-led households in the upper quartiles.

COVID-19 has left devastation on health care and the economy around the world. Asian economies were the original epicentres of the epidemic, but they also proved to be more adept at curbing the virus's spread than other regions of the world. Fang (2021) examined some of the fast-growing literature on the pandemic's impact on labour markets, both in terms of labour demand and how work was done during this pandemic. She also looked at the effects on global supply chains, retail digitization, and a variety of government stimulus programmes (Fang, 2021). The fight against the disease in the PRC and around the world is far from over. Due to the strict contact tracing the PRC government implemented, only those who did not show any symptoms and had not been in contact of anyone testing positive in the preceding 14 days were allowed to move, and all domestic cross-city travellers had to undergo a 14-day quarantine (later reduced to seven days) (Fang, 2021).

Fang and colleagues (2020) explored empirically how the COVID-19 pandemic affected labour demand across a number of cities in the PRC, whereas Dai et al. (2020) used survey data to summarize the economic impact of the COVID-19 pandemic. Using a web-scraping technique, they acquired data on job postings made between January 1st, 2018, and April 30th, 2020, on one of the PRC's most popular online platforms for hiring services. All of these factors were taken into consideration when writing each ad: location, number of open positions (if any), name and size of the company (if any), industry categorization (if any). Their sample gathered about 20 million job advertisements total, with 104.9 million job opportunities published by more than 700,000 businesses (Fang, 2021; Fang & Yeung, 2020).

Politicians have politicized the COVID-19 epidemic in order to gain political mileage over their opponents. It increases the likelihood of the virus spreading as well as the higher social costs of putting preventive measures in place. At the beginning of the pandemic, it looked as though we could transcend politics. That was obviously the first step. That spirit, however, did not endure (Hohman, 2020). The United States, for example, follows a similar playbook and adjusts its responses based on its assessment of the pandemic's severity. Whether they aim to be tighter or not, Republican governors tighten rules when situations appear to be deteriorating, and Democratic governors reduce restrictions when conditions appear to be improving (Ullah & Huque, 2020). Each governor must make difficult decisions regarding how to act. Democrats may demand tighter restrictions, while Republicans desire increased reopening, but it all comes down to the margins (Hohman, 2020).

When our behaviour is influenced by interwoven personal ties, politics enters the picture. Individuals identify with those with whom they identify, and politics is one of the factors that divides people into groups. If one individual believes we should be exceedingly cautious while another believes we should be less cautious, their behaviour will be affected. Republicans are being less cautious, while Democrats are being more cautious, now that the pandemic has become a political issue. Both of these traits may have negative consequences. Excessive caution increases the risk of the infection spreading and causing direct damage. Indirect harm, such as lost profits and income, uncertainty about when things will return to normal, and the stress associated with implementing potential solutions, will also increase. Excessive caution extends the duration of indirect injury (Hohman, 2020).

The International Monetary Fund (IMF) predicts that China's GDP will grow by 8.1 percent in 2021. Although this would still be above the global average of 5.5 percent, it would drastically reduce the discrepancy between the PRC and the rest of the world's growth (Huang et al., 2021). A significant shift in market mood could occur if the global economy continues to grow at its current pace. More crucially, in terms of economic development, China's economy confronts enormous challenges in 2021.

A number of issues for digital technologies and automation flow from the epidemic's failure to make people work from home. Remote employment can be made possible by technology, but not all industries use it in the same manner. The COVID-19 outbreak has had a significant impact on the global labour market. A vast number of occupations have been radically reshaped as a result. Businesses have been compelled to close or reduce staffing levels, which has resulted in a rise in the number of persons seeking unemployment insurance (UI) benefits (Petropoulos, 2021a). Preliminary assessments show that the pandemic's short-term effects will directly impact labour markets and employment. OECD (2020a) shows that the United States' unemployment rate rose to 14.7 percent in April 2020. Since February 2020 (as opposed to 3.5 percent) in September 2020, the rate is expected to be 7.90 percent. Unemployment rose from 2.4 percent in February 2020 to 3 percent in August 2020, despite the COVID-19 pandemic having a reduced impact on Japan's unemployment rate (Petropoulos, 2021a).

Work from home or from a remote location appears to be more successful and productive. Many jobs in the service industry are inextricably linked to these activities and cannot be totally replicated by automated systems and artificial intelligence if remote labour is completely replaced by office time or business travel twenty-one years from now (Petropoulos, 2021a). In light of the pandemic's long-term impact on low-skilled employees, Petropoulos (2021b) examine this concept: For people who spend a significant amount of time away from their homes for work, many occupations relevant to their needs are experiencing sharp declines in demand. These include construction and cleaning services; hotel and restaurant staff; urban transportation services (taxi and ride-hailing drivers); and many more. More over a quarter of all workers in the United States are employed by these services. Major job losses and a drastic shift in the labour market are expected as a result of a long-term decline in demand.

By investing in the repair and restoration of corporations, governments may reinvigorate their economies. On the other hand, developing countries are unable to do so and face a hefty repair bill as a result of their lack of funds. The poorest countries should negotiate lower payments to foreign creditors, including private borrowers, in order to increase public spending. By committing to fiscal viability in the long run, for example, through mandatory debt reduction targets, the rest should strengthen public borrowing capability. Overspending should be curtailed, and assets controlled by the government wherever possible, and all but a portion of the money should be spent to repair the business (Rajan, 2021).

In order for COVID recovery and SDG implementation to be successful, government aid must not put democratic institutions and norms at risk. There are widespread claims that COVID-19 appears being used as a pretext to suspend democratic institutions that serve as checks and balances against authoritarian power grabs in some nations (Olsen et al., 2021).

New vaccinations are being developed at a rapid pace thanks to government funds totalling billions of dollars. As a result, they already exist, but there is no worldwide immunization programme in place to ensure their equal distribution (Ullah et al., 2021). To put an end to the pandemic's devastating economic and societal effects, vaccine development technology should be made widely available (Unmüßig & Alexandra, 2021). In addition, it would serve as a powerful symbol of worldwide solidarity and cooperation.

First in the United States and then in Europe, vaccination egoism was gaining traction. Developed economies buy their medicines and demand disproportionate fees from pharmaceutical companies for new vaccine patents. This, on the other hand, hinders the ability of emerging markets to build the industrial capacity that they require. Russia, China, and India will have a long-term impact on us as a result of their strategic strength (Paul et al., 2021; Unmüßig & Alexandra, 2021).

There is an obvious disparity in immunization delivery between aspiration and reality. Since its inception, efforts to combat the COVID-19 epidemic have relied heavily on cooperation. Borrel (2020) cautioned in March 2020 that "a global pandemic needs global measures, and Europe must lead the way." An international framework for its containment was really established as soon as the epidemic began. With the ACT Accelerator set to go live on April 1, 2020, the World Health Organization (WHO), the European Commission (EC), and the French government hoped to bring governments, academia, and civil society together to make COVID-19 diagnostics and treatments, as well as vaccine development, more widely available in all countries. The goal of the COVID-19 Vaccines Global Access (COVAX) platform is to assist in the development and manufacture of COVID-19 vaccine candidates and ease cost negotiation. The primary goal is to ensure that children in developing nations receive timely access to immunizations regardless of their financial resources. It is the goal of COVAX to procure vaccine doses from manufacturers and distribute them to member countries. More than 190 countries, including 98 wealthy nations and 92 low and middle-income countries, are now covered by COVAX, with the European Union donating one billion euros (Unmüßig & Sitenko, 2021).

Unsurprisingly, extreme poverty is at the root of many of the world's worst wars, all the more so when accompanied by growing inequality. The public is aware of the connection between long-term conflict, insecurity, and poverty (Jerving, 2021). Economic inequalities and grievances are more likely to trigger conflict in South Asia (Ullah & Haque, 2020; Fleming et al., 2020; Ferdous & Ullah, 2022) than social exclusion and ethnic imbalance (Collier et al., 2009). Rising riches and innumerable technological advancements have failed to alleviate South Asia's widespread illiteracy, malnutrition, and avoidable maternal and child mortality (Akseer et al., 2017; Gani et al., 2021). Poverty perpetuates a vicious cycle of disillusionment, and conflict, exacerbated by societal injustices, caste-based marginalization, and widespread inequality.

Due to the region's history of violence and enormous inequalities, an infectious disease outbreak exploiting the region's socioeconomic vulnerability seemed inevitable. The COVID-19 pandemic highlights the region's inadequate health infrastructure, emergency planning, early disease detection, and social support networks. This has resulted in huge social and economic disruptions throughout South Asia, as well as a rise in mortality in a number of nations, including Sri Lanka, which was spared during the pandemic's early stages due to its geographical location. Millions of girls who dropped out of school ended up marrying earlier than recommended age resulting in increased adolescent pregnancy. In varied ways, an estimated 434 million children have been affected by the pandemic (Unicef, 2021).

Concerns have been expressed about the long-term impact of health-related measures on peace and stability (Rushton & McInnes, 2006). Historically, humanitarian assistance and mass vaccinations (against diseases such as smallpox and polio) have been effective in resolving wars in Africa and Latin America (de Quadros & Epstein, 2002). In South Asia, there have been moments where public health problems have trumped war, such as the tremendous outpouring of sympathy and compassion for Pakistan in 2005 and Pakistan's recent response to India's COVID-19 pandemic.

As a result, health practitioners frequently collaborate with civil society organizations and networks in their communities to promote peace, health, and well-being. Like the International Medical Doctors for the Prevention of Nuclear War and the International Campaign to Abolish nuclear weapons, several organizations have long advocated for regional peace and de-escalation (Bhutta et al., 2021). Collaboration between public health and development professionals across South Asia is critical to the region's overall progress, including education and regional security. There are numerous examples of health professionals from other countries cooperating to assist their neighbours during the calamity, and they must do the same with COVID-19 (Bhutta et al., 2021).

Southeast Asia's politics have stagnated, and democracy has weakened over the previous fifteen years. In 2020, the region averted a pandemic but is now grappling with a massive COVID-19 outbreak. While the present pandemic is wreaking havoc on individuals and the economy, it is also fuelling frustration with the political system.

Southeast Asia was the heart of a global democratic wave between 1980 and the early 2000s with democracies taking root in Indonesia, the Philippines, and Thailand, among others. Timor-Leste gained independence from Indonesia and became a democracy. Cambodia, Malaysia, and Myanmar have also experienced political reforms. Since the late 2000s, the region has been becoming politically isolated, a trend that appears to be expanding globally. For example, in Cambodia, the Philippines, and Thailand, authoritarian populists have stifled liberties. Military juntas have seized power in Thailand and Myanmar, crushing democracy. Jokowi, Indonesian

President Joko Widodo, and other professed reformers have fallen short in their efforts to eliminate corruption, hence strengthening anti-democratic organizations. Several of Asia's most despotic countries are evolving into dictatorships. The pandemic accelerated this reversal, as leaders utilized it to secure additional executive authority in the aftermath of the disease. Cambodia, Indonesia, Myanmar, Thailand, and the Philippines were ranked worse in Freedom House's 2021 worldwide freedom assessment than in its 2020 report.

Southeast Asian countries had an excellent start. COVID-19 primarily spared most Southeast Asian countries during the first year of the pandemic. Despite massive outbreaks in Indonesia and the Philippines, the number of infections remained low in Myanmar. Thai and Vietnamese leaders implemented mask use, contact tracing, border restrictions, and quarantining (Kurlantzick, 2021; Ullah, Haji-Othman & Daud, 2021). A number of factors impeded the efforts the Southeast Asian countries made to remove the virus by 2021. Some authoritarian governments first managed COVID-19 through border restrictions and other centrally controlled measures, but by 2021, the threat had evolved with introducing the more contagious Delta form. In terms of pandemic policy, countries such as Vietnam have struggled to abandon a "zero-COVID" position.

These failures are attributed to a corrupt and authoritarian government or political situations in which leaders waste their time fighting among themselves rather than addressing the disease. Due to the Thai government's initial decision to outsource vaccine production to a business controlled by the Thai king, the corporation was unable to meet demand. Myanmar's military dictatorship appears to be withholding vaccines from political opponents (Kurlantzick, 2021). For the last year, Malaysian politics has been dominated by political conflicts and pandemic-related emergency decrees, with no clear strategy in place to cope with the pandemic.

COVID-19 patients are dying in their homes in Myanmar owing to a lack of oxygen, treatment, and vaccines. Malaysia has one of the highest daily COVID-19 infection rates per capita in the world. Each day, over 1,000 new cases are reported in Thailand. Although Southeast Asian countries have recorded roughly 217,000 COVID-19 deaths since the beginning, a recent Economist analysis predicts that the genuine figure could be 2.5 to 8 times higher (Economist, 2021; Kurlantzick, 2021).

The pandemic may result in Southeast Asia's most significant political shifts since the 1990s. Even when autocrats retained power, their legitimacy decreased. Indonesians, Malaysians, Filipinos, and Thais have reached a point of desperation as a result of COVID-19's spread and economic harm. As a result, there have been increased protests. Thailand and Myanmar have recently had massive anti-government rallies, while Malaysia's government collapsed earlier in 2021, owing in part to political infighting and public dissatisfaction with government policies (Choudhury, 2021). Despite the epidemic, Singapore held elections, and the People's Action Party (PAP) was re-elected with a greater vote percentage than in the previous general election in 2010 (Kurlantzick, 2021).

Cambodia's Prime Minister, Hun Sen, has stated that he plans to remain in power for at least ten years. Indonesian President Jokowi has stated that he intends to advocate for constitutional amendments. He has, however, denied running for a third

Implications for Politics 169

term as president, thus violating Indonesia's two-term limit. Myanmar's government has proved its willingness to employ lethal force against peaceful demonstrators. Thailand's military and police have repressed dissent with ruthlessness. The virus was probably so lethal that it sparked political instability in Southeast Asian countries that are more autocratic than Brazil (Kurlantzick, 2021).

Southeast Asia's soiled regimes are abruptly confronted with a new political reality. Some Southeast Asian politicians are capable of governing force, but the vast majority are incapable. As a result, they are forced to stage elections that are not really free and fair but nonetheless allow the ruling parties to lose. Indeed, many voters in the region desire political leaders who prioritize effective public health policy over partisanship, repression, and polarization.

Citizens may be able to topple unpopular and repressive administrations. After a lengthy, high-pressure campaign, such as Malaysia's Bersih Movement, reformist voters can be consolidated around a single party or alliance during election season. Additionally, it is possible to halt democratic backsliding by protesting and mobilizing Southeast Asians to state unequivocally that they will not tolerate further destruction of institutions such as independent media, anti-corruption commissions, and impartial judiciaries by foreign democracy-promotion organizations operating in the region (Kurlantzick, 2021). Malaysia's premier reformist party has formed a coalition with the country's long-ruling party, the United Malays National Organization (UMNO), in order to govern jointly and investigate new pandemic strategies, demonstrating how this requirement for competent administration can affect regional politics. Popular support for the move is expected to be intense following a year of unproductive government. When Malaysians return to the polls, reformers will have another opportunity to grab power.

The Recovery Plans

Is resilience the Only Option?

Bottom 10 percent income has risen by slightly more than twice since 1980, despite the fact that top 1 percent income has increased by more than fourfold. A decade prior to and a decade post-global financial crisis, top 10 percent of earners had a greater share than the bottom 50 percent of earners (Huang & Saxena, 2021). The absence of redistributive policies further worsened inequality. Middle- and low-income countries have generally had very modest income redistribution (Huang & Saxena, 2021). Growth prospects and poverty reduction initiatives can be negatively impacted by persistent and rising inequality, such as raising the likelihood of a crisis or making it more difficult for the poor to invest in education (Berg & Ostry, 2011). Even in countries with low per capita income, this is the case (Barro, 1999). Improving social mobility and creating social instability are two further ways inequality harms long-term prosperity (Ferreira & Schoch, 2020). Pandemics, for example, have the potential to trigger a vicious cycle of economic collapse, inequality, and social upheaval (Sedik et al., 2020).

Even if the economy has grown, it has not necessarily led to an increase in the overall quality of life. Despite the fact that all of the region's economies had a rise in GDP per capita between 2006 and 2017, the picture was less clear when it came to people's overall happiness. In about half of the countries polled in 2017, Helliwell, Layard & Sachs (2017), satisfaction levels were lower. As it turns out, there is a correlation between increased per-capita wealth and increased happiness, but only to a certain level (Layard, 2005). The fact that one's income rises quickly doesn't necessarily mean that one is happier. A quarter century ago, China's GDP grew fivefold, but its subjective well-being declined for 15 straight years before finally rebounding and remaining lower than it was in the early 1990s (World Happiness Report, 2017). In the poll, factors that contribute to happiness other than income include healthy life expectancy, trust (reported absence of corruption in government and business), perceived decision-making freedom, and generousness (recent donations) (Helliwell et al., 2017).

In 2020 and 2021, a decline in foreign travel might cost the global economy $4 trillion or more. Tourists, as well as those who work in other industries that are directly affected by the outbreak, are expected to lose money. In 2021, the tourism industry could suffer a similar loss, and its recovery will rely on how widely COVID-19 vaccines are accepted (UNCTAD, 2021). A 28 percent drop in remittances was expected due to the global coronavirus epidemic in 2020. Compared to pre-COVID-19 levels in 2019, the amount of money sent back home by migrant workers is expected to decline by 14 percent by 2021 as a result of the epidemic and economic crisis. LMIC remittances are expected to fall by 7 percent in 2020, to $508 billion, before falling further 7.5 percent in 2021 to $470 billion (World Bank, 2020).

This is a direct outcome of the pandemic's 600 million job losses (Ullah et al., 2021) implying that the unemployment rate has risen. In the worst-affected countries, business failure and poverty are especially widespread. Supply disruptions, job and income uncertainty, a range of health, security, and labour rights problems, and rising poverty are challenges for micro, small, and medium-sized firms. People in low-skilled jobs, migrants, members of racial and ethnic minorities, the elderly and those with disabilities have all been affected by this epidemic. HIV/AIDS patients have also been affected. The crisis intensified an already severe scarcity of high-quality jobs, aggravated poverty, deepened inequality, and exposed digital gaps across and among countries (ILO, 2021).

It is not unknown that several of the world's wealthiest countries hoard COVID-19 vaccines. However, in low-income nations, less than one percent of people have gotten at least one dose. With nearly 4 million deaths and huge economic losses, the pandemic appeared clearly as a global problem that necessitates a global response. Vaccine injustice not only harms people but it also exacerbates already substantial socioeconomic disparities. The pandemic's indirect effects have disproportionately impacted women and girls, ranging from a threefold rise in infection rates for female healthcare professionals compared to male colleagues to a 19 percent increase in unemployment risk (ILO, 2020). Refugees and people have also been disproportionately affected. Lower-income countries host 40 million refugees while receiving only 3 percent of the world's vaccination supply (Mansour, 2021). If attempts to distribute lifesaving vaccines are not considerably enhanced in the coming months, the consequences for such communities would be terrible. Migrant populations are the most vulnerable to the COVID-19 epidemic, and they bear the brunt of the consequences of its spread—directly as a threat to health and life, and indirectly as a result of remedies such as border restrictions and draconian lockdowns (Sengupta & Jha, 2020; Ullah et al., 2021). On 15 August 2020, migrants made up an average of 5 percent of the population in the top ten COVID-19-affected countries (UN DESA, 2019; WHO, 2020), with the United States and Spain accounting for more than 13 percent and 13 percent, respectively, compared to a global rate of 3.5 percent. The top ten COVID-19-affected countries include both emigration and immigration destinations: the US, Russia, and Spain all have sizable international migration populations, while India, Mexico, and Brazil are significant senders (Yadav, 2021).

The vast majority of epidemiological studies have been undertaken in developed countries and politically stable developing countries. Armed conflict has a complicated and diversified impact on the prevalence of infectious diseases (DAW, 2021). Rarely have investigations on the impact of war on COVID-19 transmission in conflict zones been done. This was amply demonstrated in Africa during the Ebola outbreak. Physical violence involving at least one organized group have killed an average of more than 105,000 people every year over the last six years (Pettersson & Öberg, 2020). Armed conflict substantially negatively influences human security and effectively represents "reverse progress" (Ide, 2021). However, contradictory findings have been found regarding both increases and decreases in infectious disease transmission during and after wars (DAW, 2021). It is vital to assess the impact of COVID-19 on armed conflict, with a focus on its most common form, intrastate armed conflict. The previous study confirms that infectious diseases directly impact the start and duration of armed conflicts. Economic decline and poor health are also the predictors of civil strife. Increased intensity of armed conflict jeopardizes efforts to contain the pandemic (Mehrl & Thurner, 2020) because armed groups mistakenly or deliberately destroy infrastructure vital for a healthy lifestyle, such as water, electricity, and health services delivery. In line with this, we find that high-intensity armed conflict increased the death rate of female non-combatants in Africa by 202 percent (Fiedler et al., 2021; Ide, 2021; Manley & Steinberg, 2020).

Only a few of the elements fuelling the epidemic are societal divisions, serious disruptions in the educational system, and worsening economic challenges. Furthermore, the epidemic has dramatically lowered the number of people and organizations capable of preventing violence. As a result of unhappiness with how the pandemic was handled, many governments' and security agencies' trust in their governments has plummeted (Fiedler et al., 2021).

COVID-19 flew from Wuhan, China, to Europe and other nations with significant international trade hubs and migrant populations. The pandemic gradually spread to other continents, including Africa, East Asia, and Western Asia. As the virus spread across migrant-receiving countries, workers, international students, asylum seekers, and refugees became increasingly vulnerable (Truelove et al., 2020). As the situation worsened, many international migrants returned to India, Pakistan, and Bangladesh, notably those from Gulf Cooperation Council (GCC) nations. In addition, there were significant returns to Afghanistan from Iran (150,000) and Pakistan (60,000) (BBC, 2020). The Indian government's shutdown has substantially impacted the lives of the country's almost 40 million internal migrants, pushing 50,000–60,000 people to relocate from metropolitan areas to rural areas of origin in a couple of days. Authorities set up camps with inadequate services in towns, transit hubs, and origin locations to shelter these people (Bindra & Sharma, 2020).

There should be no stigma or discrimination when it comes to certain COVID-19-related medical procedures like gender identity and sexual orientation. As a result of public awareness initiatives, everyone now has access to free healthcare. In order to ensure that vulnerable people seeking lifesaving care do not fear deportation or reprisal, governments should take steps to construct barriers between healthcare practitioners and illegal migrants, particularly when it comes to COVID-19 testing or therapy. Due to financial restrictions, governments contend that people should not be denied COVID-19 testing, treatment, or care. As in the United States, an additional 28 million individuals lack health insurance, and even if they are covered, more than a quarter of patients cannot afford care. Because of the high cost of medical treatment and prescription medications, many Americans are concerned about their health. Avoiding medical attention during an outbreak is detrimental to people who are ill and accelerates the spread of the coronavirus. All countries commit to take actions to prevent a serious public health problem from turning into a human rights tragedy due to people's inability to get proper medical care. Governments must take steps to guarantee that all inhabitants have easy access to affordable health care (Human Rights Watch, 2020).

Let's Not This Pandemic Go To Waste

Today, global prosperity and quality of life are clearly threatened by COVID-19, which reduces the chance of achieving the SDGs. Even in the midst of a crisis, there are audible and hopeful voices who recognize that possibilities may arise (Duek & Fliss, 2020). An opportunity is opening up for countries to move away from "business as usual" and toward more sustainable growth paths. One of the most critical aspects of this transformation is the inclusion of new funding and behavioural adjustments (Olsen et al., 2021).

Environmentalists have a glimmer of hope because of the pandemic. There has been a reduction in air pollution worldwide as a result of governments' worldwide shelter-in-place directives resulting in fewer traffic, reduced air travel, and lower industry emissions. Particularly beneficial for lung health in this situation, the air quality is better than it has been in certain regions for decades. Shelter-in-place orders may encourage environmental laws and regulations that would eventually lead to better air, despite experts' warnings (Preira, 2020). To combat a pandemic, we need increased coordination and multi-sectoral cooperation as a society committed to a common destiny for humanity in order to respond promptly and prevent the disease from spreading rapidly (Sullivan et al., 2020). Our priority sets for exchanging information and data, research priorities, and global pandemic surveillance and response must be quickly upgraded in collaboration with more international partners.

Certain nations, such as India, have had extremely high rates of Covid-19 infection, having a severe impact on population health as well as social and economic well-being (Babu et al., 2021). In other parts of the world, such as Israel, where around 90 percent of the population has received two doses of the vaccine, the illness has been successfully managed. Vaccine development, like the development of many previous pharmaceutical products, is reliant on government funding of universities, pharmaceutical laboratories, and for-profit pharmaceutical businesses. Despite the fact that the majority of early research takes place in universities, pharmaceutical companies have the resources, expertise, and experience necessary to move medical breakthroughs from the laboratory to clinical trials, regulatory approval, and finally to doctors or pharmacists who can administer them (Gupta & Baru, 2020).

Global vaccination market revenues are dominated by high-income countries, but they make up just 16 percent of the world's population and account for less than 6 percent of all infectious disease-related deaths (20 percent by number of vaccines). There is a movement in the global vaccine market and innovation toward people in high-demand regions. With the help of UNICEF, GAVI, the Vaccine Alliance, is able to provide immunizations to children in some of the world's poorest countries. GAVI-funded immunizations were given to up to 65 million children in 2019 (Economicsobservatory, 2020).

Governments at all levels of international collaboration are involved. They may fund basic research, whereas vaccines are frequently purchased as a result of this. In a way, governments function as both investors and buyers. Finally, the vaccination market is extremely consolidated on both sides of the aisle. As a result, only a few corporations manufacture vaccines, and even fewer individuals purchase them. Four corporations dominated the global vaccine market in 2019, but COVID-19 has altered that dynamic. Vaccines that have lost their patent protection are often produced by generic pharmaceutical companies. Any pharmaceutical business may develop a drug or vaccine if it can demonstrate that the product is safe. This enhances competition, in contrast to when vaccines are patent-protected, in which the firm that developed them retains exclusive rights to manufacture them. As a result, the vast majority of vaccines that are no longer patent-protected across the world have low prices and profit margins.

The world cannot afford a new cold war or a division. We must accept the fact that no country is safe is every country is not safe. Hence, vaccine equity must be ensured. Hoarding vaccine does not demonstrate power; rather, it causes divisiveness. A virus is not politics. Let no country be used as a scapegoat. This is an opportunity for all wealthy countries to demonstrate that humanity transcends all forms of politics and commerce.

174   5 Choosing to End the Pandemic: Conclusions and Discussion

As of February 27, 2022, the number of Coronavirus cases has climbed to 436,148,210, with 5,969,147 deaths and 366,731,850 recoveries. COVID-19, on the other hand, is no longer generating headlines since the Russia-Ukraine crisis erupted. After diplomatic attempts failed, Russian troops advanced on Ukraine in late February 2022. Just a few months after taking office, the Biden administration spoke of a "strong, predictable" relationship with Russia. That appears to be out of the question at the moment. The White House has issued sanctions against Russia, and the US is supplying money and weapons to Ukraine while also strengthening its military presence in Europe. European leaders have met with Russian President Vladimir Putin one-on-one in recent weeks.

Another factor that could affect military planning for the Russian and Ukrainian militaries is the emergence of Covid, as record numbers of cases are duplicated among the personnel in both countries. Thousands of soldiers are infected with the disease while on active duty. Visitors have been prevented from entering Ukrainian military locations in an attempt to halt the spread of the disease. Covid may have infected Russian troops stationed near the border or participating in military manoeuvres in Belarus. Ukraine's health ministry has reported 43,778 new cases since the outbreak began, the most in a single day since the outbreak began. There was an almost 4,000 increases over the previous day. Russia has also been heavily affected by the Omicron variety, with 168,201 new infections reported in the previous 24 h (Anand, 2022), an all-time high on February 25th, 2022. The global politics has replaced the global pandemic in news headlines.

References

Akseer, N., Kamali, M., Arifeen, S. E., Malik, A., Bhatti, Z., Thacker, N., Maksey, M., D'Silva, H., Da Silva, I. C. M., & Bhutta, Z. A. (2017). Progress in maternal and child health: How has South Asia fared? *BMJ, 357.*

Anand, J. C. (2022, February 25). *Russia-Ukraine crisis: India among worst losers in Asia.* https://economictimes.indiatimes.com/news/economy/indicators/russia-ukraine-crisis-india-among-worst-losers-in-asia-report-says/articleshow/89817187.cms

Ashford, E., & Kroenig, M. (2020, March 20). *How will the Coronavirus pandemic reshape the U.S. election?* https://foreignpolicy.com/2020/03/20/how-will-coronavirus-pandemic-reshape-2020-us-election/. Accessed 7 Aug 2021.

Babu, G. R., Khetrapal, S., John, D. A., Deepa, R., & Narayan, K. M. V. (2021). Pandemic preparedness and response to COVID-19 in South Asian countries. *International Journal of Infectious Diseases, 105*, 169–174.

Barro, R. J. (1999). *Inequality, growth, and investment* (NBER Working Paper 7038). National Bureau of Economic Research. www.nber.org/system/files/working_papers/w7038/w7038.pdf. Accessed 10 July 2021.

BBC. (2020, June 23). Millions become millionaires during Covid pandemic. *BBC News.* https://www.bbc.com/news/business-57575077. Accessed 12 July 2021.

Berg, A. G., & Ostry, J. D. (2011). *Inequality and unsustainable growth: Two sides of the same coin?* (IMF Staff Discussion Note No. SDN/11/08). International Monetary Fund. www.imf.org/external/pubs/ft/sdn/2011/sdn1108.pdf

References

Betancourt, J. A., Rosenberg, M. A., Zevallos, A., Brown, J. R., & Mileski, M. (2020). The impact of COVID-19 on telemedicine utilization across multiple service lines in the United States. *Healthcare (Basel, Switzerland), 8*(4), 380. https://doi.org/10.3390/healthcare8040380

Bhutta, Z. A., Mitra, A., Salman, A., Akbari, F., Dalil, S., Jehan, F., Chowdhury, M., Jayasinghe, S., Menon, P., Nundy, S., Qadri, F., Islam, M. T., & & Gautam, K. (2021). Conflict, extremism, resilience and peace in South Asia; can covid-19 provide a bridge for peace and rapprochement? *BMJ, 375*, e067384.

Bindra, J., & Sharma, N. C. (2020). *Coronavirus: Govt tells SC one-third of migrant workers could be infected*. https://www.livemint.com/news/india/covid-19-govt-tells-sc-one-third-of-migrant-wor kers-could-be-infected-11585643185390.html

Bolleyer, N., & Salát, O. (2021). Parliaments in times of crisis: COVID-19, populism and executive dominance. *West European Politics, 44*(5–6), 1103–1128.

Borrel, J. (2020). *EU HRVP Josep Borrell: The Coronavirus pandemic and the new world it is creating*. https://eeas.europa.eu/delegations/china/76401/eu-hrvp-josep-borrell-coronavirus-pan demic-and-new-world-it-creating_en. Accessed 13 July 2021.

Calisher, C., Carroll, D., Colwell, R., Corley, R. B., Daszak, P., Drosten, C., Enjuanes, L., Farrar, J., Field, H., Golding, J., Gorbalenya, A., Haagmans, B., Hughes, J. M., Karesh, W. B., Keusch, G. T., Lam, S. K., Lubroth, J., Mackenzie, J. S., Madoff, L., Mazet, J., Palese, P., Perlman, S., Poon, L., Roizman, B., Saif, L., Subbarao., & Turner, M. (2020). Statement in support of the scientists, public health professionals, and medical professionals of China combatting COVID-19. *The Lancet, 395*(10226), e42–e43.

Choudhury, S. R. (2021, August 9). Charts show that Covid is hitting parts of Asia harder now than when the pandemic began. *CNBC*. https://www.cnbc.com/2021/08/10/covid-is-hitting-parts-of-asia-harder-now-than-beginning-of-pandemic.html. Accessed 10 Oct 2021.

Collier, P., Hoeffler, A., & Rohner, D. (2009). Beyond greed and grievance: Feasibility and civil war. *Oxford Economic Papers, 61*(1), 1–27.

Congressional Research Service (CRS). (2021). *Global economic effects of COVID-19*. Congressional Research Service. https://fas.org/sgp/crs/row/R46270.pdf. Accessed 30 July 2021.

DAW, M. A. (2021). The impact of armed conflict on the epidemiological situation of Coronavirus disease (COVID-19) in Libya, Syria, and Yemen. Mohamed A Daw. *Frontiers in Public Health, 9*, 698.

De Quadros, C. A., & Epstein, D. (2002). Health as a bridge for peace: PAHO's experience. *The Lancet, 360*, s25–s26.

Dionne, K., & Turkmen, F. (2020). The politics of pandemic othering: Putting COVID-19 in global and historical context. *International Organization, 74*(S1), E213–E230. https://doi.org/10.1017/ S0020818320000405

Dollar, D. (2020, November 17). The future of global supply chains: What are the implications for international trade? *Brookings*. https://www.brookings.edu/research/the-future-of-global-sup ply-chains-what-are-the-implications-for-international-trade/. Accessed 30 July 2021.

Economicsobservatory. (2020). *How does the market for vaccines work?* https://www.economics observatory.com/how-does-the-market-for-vaccines-work. Accessed 23 Dec 2021.

Economist. (2021, January 9). *What is the economic cost of Covid-19?* https://www.econom ist.com/finance-and-economics/2021/01/09/what-is-the-economic-cost-of-covid-19. Accessed 7 Aug 2020.

Eiran, E. (2020). *COVID-19 and great power rivalry*. http://sam.gov.tr/pdf/sam-yayinlari/The% 20World%20after%20COVID19.pdf. Accessed 30 July 2021.

Fang, H., & Yeung, B. (2020). Post–COVID-19 reconfiguration of the global value chains and China. In S. Agarwal, Z. He, & B. Yeung (Eds.), *Impact of COVID-19 on Asian economies and policy responses* (pp. 151–156). https://www.worldscientific.com/doi / https://doi.org/10.1142/ 9789811229381_0021

Fang, H., Ge, C., Huang, H., & Li, H. (2020). *Pandemics, global supply chains, and local labor demand: Evidence from 100 million posted jobs in China* (No. w28072). National Bureau of Economic Research.

Fang, H. (2021). COVID-19: The impact on the economy and policy responses—A review. In J. Beirne, P. J. Morgan, & T. Sonobe (Eds.), *COVID-19 impacts and policy options: An Asian perspective* (pp. 281–310). Asian Development Bank.

Ferdous, J., & Ullah, A. K. M. A. (2022). COVID-19 and migrant population in South Asia: Exploring the resilience. *IJAPS, 18*(2).

Ferreira, F., & Schoch, M. (2020, February 24). Inequality and social unrest in Latin America: The Tocqueville paradox revisited. *World Bank Blog*. https://blogs.worldbank.org/developmenttalk/inequality-and-social-unrest-latin-america-tocqueville-paradox-revisited. Accessed 2 May 2021.

Fiedler, C., Mross, K., & Adeto, Y. (2021). Conflict and peace. In J. Leininger, C. Strupat, Y. Adeto, A. Shimeles, W. Wasike, M. Aleksandrova, C. Brandi, M. Brüntrup, F. Burchi, E. Dick, & A. Berger (Eds.), *The COVID-19 pandemic and structural transformation in Africa: Evidence for action* (Discussion Paper 11/2021). German Development Institute / Deutsches Institut für Entwicklungspolitik (DIE).

Flanagan, R. (2021, July 21). Why is Canada outpacing the U.S. in vaccinations? *CTV News*. https://www.ctvnews.ca/health/coronavirus/why-is-canada-outpacing-the-u-s-in-vaccinations-fauci-says-we-don-t-have-their-divisiveness-1.5517600. Accessed 11 May 2021.

Fleming, C. M., Manning, M., Pham, H. T., & Vorsina, M. (2020). Ethnic economic inequality and fatalities from terrorism. *Journal of iIterpersonal Violence*, 0886260520976226.

Flinders, M. (2021). Democracy and the politics of coronavirus: Trust, blame and understanding. *Parliamentary Affairs, 74*(2), 483–502.

Freedman, P. (2019). *American cuisine: And how it got this way*. Liveright.

Gani, M. S., Ullah, A. K. M., A., Subramaniam, T., Nyström, L., Chowdhury, A., & Mushtaque, R. (2021). Reduction in lifetime fertility from BRAC's maternal neonatal and child survival intervention in rural Bangladesh. *Asia Pacific Journal of Rural Development, 31*(2), 1–15.

Glosserman, B. (2020, March 11). Fighting COVID-19: It's the story, stupid. *The Japan Times*. https://www.japantimes.co.jp/opinion/2020/03/11/commentary/japan-commentary/fighting-covid-19-story-stupid/

Government of Bangladesh (GoB). (2020). *COVID-19: Bangladesh multi-sectoral anticipatory impact and needs analysis*. https://reliefweb.int/sites/reliefweb.int/files/resources/COVID_NAWG%20Anticipatory%20Impacts%20and%20Needs%20Analysis.pdf. Accessed 2 Aug 2021.

Guadagno, L. (2020). *Migrants and the COVİD-19 pandemic: An initial analysis* (Migration Research Series, No. 60). International Organization for Migration.

Gunther, A. (2020). COVID-19: Fight or flight. *Agriculture and Human Values, 1–2*. https://www.ncbi.nlm.nih.gov/pmc/articles/PMC7220582/

Gupta, I., & Baru, R. (2020). Economics & ethics of the COVID-19 vaccine: How prepared are we? *Indian Journal of Medical Research, 152*(1 & 2), 153–155. https://doi.org/10.4103/ijmr.IJMR_3581_20. PMID: 32896834; PMCID: PMC7853278.

Helliwell, J. F., Huang, H., & Wang, S. (2017). *World happiness report 2017*. Sustainable Development Solutions Network. https://worldhappiness.report/ed/2017/. Accessed 12 Oct 21.

Helliwell, J., Layard, R., & Sachs, J. (2017). *World happiness report 2017*. https://s3.amazonaws.com/happiness-report/2017/HR17.pdf

Hohman, J. M. (2020). Political fights make the pandemic response worse. *The Hill*. https://thehill.com/opinion/healthcare/513842-political-fights-make-the-pandemic-response-worse?rl=1. Accessed 29 July 2021.

Huang, Y., Qiu, H., & Wang, J. (2021). Digital technology and economic impacts of COVID-19: Experiences of the people's Republic of China. In J. Beirne, P. J. Morgan, & T. Sonobe (Eds.), *COVID-19 impacts and policy options: An Asian perspective* (pp. 310–335). Asian Development Bank.

Huang, Z., & Saxena, S. C. (2021). Building forward better: Enhancing the resilience of Asia and Pacific economies in a post-COVID-19 world. In J. Beirne, P. J. Morgan, & T. Sonobe (Eds.), *COVID-19 Impacts and policy options: An Asian perspective* (pp. 473–519). Asian Development Bank.

References 177

Human Rights Watch. (2020, March 19). *Human rights dimensions of COVID-19 response*. https://www.hrw.org/news/2020/03/19/human-rights-dimensions-covid-19-response#_Toc35446577. Accessed 13 July 2021.

Ide, T. (2021). COVID-19 and armed conflict. *World Development, 140*, 105355. https://doi.org/10.1016/j.worlddev.2020.105355. Accessed 10 July 2021.

International Labour Organization (ILO). (2020). *COVID-19 and the world of work* (1st ed.).

International Labour Organization (ILO). (2021). *Resolution concerning a global call to action for a human-centred recovery from the COVID-19 crisis that is inclusive, sustainable and resilient*. International Labour Conference—109th Session.

Irfan, U. (2021). *Why are rich countries still monopolizing Covid-19 vaccines?* https://www.vox.com/22759707/covid-19-vaccine-gap-covax-rich-poor-countries-boosters. Accessed 25 Dec 2021.

Jerving, S. (2021, May 10). India crisis puts Covax 150 million doses behind schedule. *Devex*. https://www.devex.com/news/india-crisis-puts-covax-150-million-doses-behind-schedule-99860. Accessed 1 Dec 2021.

Joob, B., & Wiwanitkit, V. (2020). COVID-19 and migrant workers: Lack of data and need for specific management. *Public Health, 183*, 64.

Klaus, S., & Christine, L. (2021). *Christine Lagarde on how to address COVID-19, climate change and inequality*. https://www.weforum.org/agenda/2021/09/klaus-schwab-christine-lagarde-covid-19-climate-change-inequality/

Kurlantzick, J. (2021, October 6). *Is COVID-19 shaking up politics in Southeast Asia?* Council on Foreign Relations. https://www.cfr.org/article/covid-19-shaking-politics-southeast-asia. Accessed 11 Dec 2021.

Kurz, H. D. (2017). Is there a "Ricardian Vice"? And what is its relationship with economic policy ad "vice"? *Journal of Evolutionary Economics, 27*(1), 91–114.

Layard, R. (2005). *Happiness: Lessons from a new Science*. Allen Lane.

Manley, C., & Steinberg, F. (2020, November 11). The geopolitical implications of the COVID-19 pandemic and the role of the EU in the world. *Global Spectator*. https://blog.realinstitutoelcano.org/en/the-geopolitical-implications-of-the-covid-19-pandemic-and-the-role-of-the-eu-in-the-world/. Accessed 4 Aug 2021.

Mansour, M. (2021, July 21). *How unequal COVID-19 vaccine distribution is exacerbating global inequalities*. https://www.one.org/international/blog/covid19-vaccine-inequity/. Accessed 7 Aug 2021.

McNamara, K. R., & Newman, A. L. (2020). The big reveal: COVID-19 and globalization's great transformations. *International Organization, 74*(S1), E59–E77.

Mehrl, M., & Thurner, P. W. (2020). The effect of the COVID-19 pandemic on global armed conflict: Early evidence. *Political Studies Review, 19*(2), 286–293.

Mogaji, E. (2021). Marketing the COVID-19 vaccine and the implications for public health. *Vaccine, 39*(34), 4766–4768. https://doi.org/10.1016/j.vaccine.2021.07.015

Morgan, P. J., & Trinh, L. Q. (2021). Impacts of COVID-19 on households in ASEAN countries and their implications for human capital development. In J. Beirne, P. J. Morgan, & S. Tetsushi (Eds.), *COVID-19 impacts and policy options: An Asian perspective* (pp. 188–245). Asian Development Bank.

Nicola, M., Alsafi, Z., Sohrabi, C., Kerwan, A., Al-Jabir, A., Iosifidis, C., Agha, M., & Agha, R. (2020). The socio-economic implications of the coronavirus pandemic (COVID-19): A review. *International journal of surgery, 78*, 185–193.

OECD. (2020a, November 10). *The territorial impact of COVID-19: Managing the crisis across levels of government*. OECD. https://www.oecd.org/coronavirus/policy-responses/the-territorial-impact-of-covid-19-managing-the-crisis-across-levels-of-government-d3e314e1/. Accessed 9 Mar 2021.

OECD. (2020b, November). *Unemployment rates, OECD—Updated*. https://www.oecd.org/sdd/labour-stats/unemployment-rates-oecd-update-november-2020.htm. Accessed 12 Oct 2021.

OECD. (2021). *The territorial impact of COVID-19: Managing the crisis and recovery across levels of government*. https://www.oecd.org/coronavirus/policy-responses/the-territorial-impact-of-covid-19-managing-the-crisis-and-recovery-across-levels-of-government-a2c6abaf/. Accessed 7 Mar 2021.

Olsen, S. H., Zusman, E., Hengesbaugh, M., Amanuma, N., & Onoda, S. (2021). Governing the sustainable development goals in the Covid-19 era: Bringing back hierarchic styles of governance? In J. Beirne, P. J. Morgan Peter, & T. Sonobe. (Eds.), *COVID-19 impacts and policy options: An Asian perspective* (pp. 520–544). Asian Development Bank.

Paul, B., Patnaik, U., Murari, K. K., Sahu, S. K., & Muralidharan, T. (2021). The impact of COVID-19 on the household economy of India. *The Indian Journal of Labour Economics, 64*, 867–882. https://doi.org/10.1007/s41027-021-00352-8

Perthes, V. (2020, March 31). *The Corona crisis and international relations: Open questions, tentative assumptions*. German Institute for International and Security Affairs. https://www.swp-berlin.org/en/publication/the-corona-crisis-and-international-relations-open-questions-tentative-assumptions. Accessed 30 July 2021.

Petropoulos, G. (2021a). Automation, COVID-19, and labor markets. In J. Beirne, P. J. Morgan, & T. Sonobe (Eds.), *COVID-19 impacts and policy options: An Asian perspective* (pp. 336–361). Asian Development Bank.

Petropoulos, G. (2021b). Automation, COVID-19, and labor markets. *ADBI Working Paper 1229*. Asian Development Bank Institute. Available: https://www.adb.org/publications/automation-covid-19-and-labor-markets

Pettersson, T., Högbladh, S., & Öberg, M. (2019). Organized violence, 1989–2018 and peace agreements. *Journal of Peace Research, 56*(4), 589–603.

Pettersson, T., & Öberg, M. (2020). Organized violence 1989–2019. *Journal of Peace Research, 57*(4), 597–613.

Politico. (2020, March 3). *Coronavirus will change the world permanently*. Here's How. https://www.politico.com/news/magazine/2020/03/19/coronavirus-effect-economy-life-society-analysis-covid-135579. Accessed 5 Feb 2021.

Preira, I. (2020, April 22). Cleaner air due to coronavirus pandemic makes Earth day 50th anniversary celebration bittersweet for environmentalists. *ABC NEWS*. https://abcnews.go.com/Health/cleaner-air-coronavirus-precautions-makes-earth-day-celebration/story?id=69923658. Accessed 3 Feb 2021.

Rajan, R. (2021). Dealing with corporate distress, repair, and reallocation after the pandemic. In J. Beirne, P. J. Morgan, & T. Sonobe (Eds.),*COVID-19 impacts and policy options: An Asian perspective* (pp. 385–398). Asian Development Bank.

Rothgerber, H., Wilson, T., Whaley, D., Rosenfeld, D. L., Humphrey, M., Moore, A., & Bihl, A. (2020). *Politicizing the COVID-19 pandemic: Ideological differences in adherence to social distancing*. https://doi.org/10.31234/osf.io/k23cv. pmid:31707073. Accessed 17 Feb 2021.

Rushton, S., & McInnes, C. (2006). The UK, health and peace-building: The mysterious disappearance of health as a bridge for peace. *Medicine, Conflict and Survival, 22*(2), 94–109.

Sakamoto, H., Rahman, M., Nomura, S., Okamoto, E., Koike, S., et al. (2018). *Japan health system review*. World Health Organization. Regional Office for South-East Asia. https://apps.who.int/iris/handle/10665/259941. License: CC BY-NC-SA 3.0 IGO.

Sánchez-Páramo, C., Hill, R., Mahler, D. G., Narayan, A., & Yonzan, N. (2021, October 7). *COVID-19 leaves a legacy of rising poverty and widening inequality*. World Bank. https://blogs.worldbank.org/developmenttalk/covid-19-leaves-legacy-rising-poverty-and-widening-inequality. Accessed 21 Nov 2021.

Sands, P. (2020, March 7). *COVID-19 threatens the poor and marginalized more than anyone*. https://reliefweb.int/report/world/covid-19-threatens-poor-and-marginalized-more-anyone. Accessed 21 Oct 2021.

Scudellari, M. (2020, August 5). How the pandemic might play out in 2021 and beyond. *Nature*. https://www.nature.com/articles/d41586-020-02278-5. Accessed 12 Dec 2021.

References

Sedik, T. S., Xu, R., & Stuart, A. (2020). *A vicious cycle: How pandemics lead to economic despair and social unrest* (IMF Working Papers, 2020 [216]). www.imf.org/en/Publications/WP/Issues/2020/10/16/A-Vicious-Cycle-How-Pandemics-Lead-to-Economic-Despair-and-Social-Unrest-49806. Accessed 12 Dec 2021.

Sengupta, S., & Jha, M. K. (2020). Social policy, COVID-19 and impoverished migrants: Challenges and prospects in locked down India. *The International Journal of Community and Social Development, 2*(2), 152–172. https://doi.org/10.1177/2516602620933715

Shang, Y., Li, H., & Zhang, R. (2021). Effects of pandemic outbreak on economies: Evidence From business history context. *Frontiers in Public Health, 9*, 146–150.

Siche, R. (2020). What is the impact of COVID-19 disease on agriculture? *Scientia Agropecuaria, 11*(1), 3–6.

Stigler, G. J. (1952). The Ricardian theory of value and distribution. *Journal of Political Economy, 60*(3), 187–207. http://www.jstor.org/stable/1826451

Sullivan, A. D., Strickland, C. J., & Howard, K. M. (2020). Public health emergency preparedness practices and the management of frontline communicable disease response. *Journal of Public Health Management and Practice, 26*(2), 180–183.

The Japan Times. (2020). *Have we learned enough from the 1995 Kobe quake?* https://www.japantimes.co.jp/opinion/2020/01/16/editorials/learned-enough-1995-kobe-quake/. Accessed 9 Jan 2021.

Torero, M. (2020). Prepare food systems for a long-haul fight against COVID-19. In J. Swinnen & J. McDermott (Eds.), *COVID-19 and global food security. Part Seven: Preparing food systems for future pandemics* (Chapter 27, pp. 118–121). International Food Policy Research Institute (IFPRI). https://doi.org/10.2499/p15738coll2.133762_27

Truelove, S., Abrahim, O., Altare, C., Lauer, S. A., Grantz, K. H., Azman, A. S., et al. (2020). The potential impact of COVID-19 in refugee camps in Bangladesh and beyond: A modeling study. *PLoS Med, 17*(6), e1003144. https://doi.org/10.1371/journal.pmed.1003144

UNCTAD. (2021, June 30). *Global economy could lose over $4 trillion due to COVID-19 impact on tourism.* https://unctad.org/news/global-economy-could-lose-over-4-trillion-due-covid-19-impact-tourism. Accessed 8 Aug 2021.

Ullah, A. A., Hossain, M. A., & Islam, K. M. (2015). *Migrants and workers fatalities.* Palgrave McMillan.

Ullah, A. A., & Haque, M. S. (2020). *The migration myth in policy and practice: Dreams, development and despair.* Springer.

Ullah, A. K. M. A., & Huque, A. S. (2020). Demoralization-led migration in Bangladesh: A sense of insecurity-based decision-making model. *Asian Journal of Comparative Politics, 5*(4), 351–370. https://doi.org/10.1177/2057891119867140

Ullah, A. K. M., Hossain, M. A., Azizuddin, M., & Nawaz, F. (2020a). Social research methods: Migration in perspective. *Migration Letters, 17*(2), 357–368.

Ullah, A. A., Hossain, M. A., & Chattoraj, D. (2020b). Covid-19 and Rohingya refugee camps in Bangladesh. *Intellectual Discourse, 28*(2), 793–806.

Ullah, A. A., Lee, S. C. W., Hassan, N. H., & Nawaz, F. (2020c). Xenophobia in the GCC countries: Migrants' desire and distress. *Global Affairs, 6*(2), 203–223.

Ullah, A. A., Hasan, N. H., Mohamad, S. M., & Chattoraj, D. (2020d). Migration and security: Implications for minority migrant groups. *India Quarterly, 76*(1), 136–153.

Ullah, A. A., Nawaz, F., & Chattoraj, D. (2021). Locked up under lockdown: The COVID-19 pandemic and the migrant population. *Social Sciences & Humanities Open, 3*(1), 100126.

Ullah, A. K. M. A., Haji-Othman, N. A., & Daud, M. K. (2021). COVID-19 and shifting border policies in Southeast Asia. *Southeast Asia: A Multidisciplinary Journal, 21*(2), 1–14.

Ullah, A. A., & Kumpoh, A. A. Z. A. (2018). Are borders the reflection of international relations? Southeast Asian borders in perspective. *Journal of Asian Security and International Affairs, 5*(3), 295–318.

Ullah, A. A., & Kumpoh, A. A. Z. A. (2019). Diaspora community in Brunei: Culture, ethnicity and integration. *Diaspora Studies, 11*(3), 14–33.

Unicef. (2021). *Racing to respond to the COVID-19 crisis in South Asia.* https://www.unicef.org/rosa/racing-respond-covid-19-crisis-south-asia. Accessed 13 Aug 2021.

Unmüßig, B., & Alexandra, S. (2021, April 1). *Divided we fail—Vaccine diplomacy and its implications.* https://hk.boell.org/en/2021/04/01/divided-we-fail-vaccine-diplomacy-and-its-implications. Accessed 16 Aug 2021.

Vogel, L., & Eggertson, L. (2020, June 12). COVID-19: A timeline of Canada's first-wave response. *CMAJ News.* https://cmajnews.com/2020/06/12/coronavirus-1095847/. Accessed 29 Aug 2021.

WHO. (2021). *2021 has been tumultuous but we know how to end the pandemic and promote health for all in 2022.* https://www.who.int/news-room/commentaries/detail/2021-has-been-tumultuous-but-we-know-how-to-end-the-pandemic-and-promote-health-for-all-in-2022

Wong, A. C. (2021, February 10). Vaccine nationalism: Rich nations must also care for the poor. *The Interpreter.* https://www.lowyinstitute.org/the-interpreter/vaccine-nationalism-rich-nations-must-also-care-poor. Accessed 24 Oct 2021.

World Bank. (2020). *Monitoring COVID-19 impacts on households in Mongolia.* https://www.worldbank.org/en/country/mongolia/brief/monitoring-covid-19-impacts-on-households-in-mongolia. Accessed 1 Aug 2021.

World Bank. (2021, June 8). *The global economy: on track for strong but uneven growth as COVID-19 still weighs.* The World Bank. https://www.worldbank.org/en/news/feature/2021/06/08/the-global-economy-on-track-for-strong-but-uneven-growth-as-covid-19-still-weighs. Accessed 5 Aug 2021.

World Economic Forum. (2021). *When will the COVID-19 pandemic end?* Experts explain. https://www.weforum.org/agenda/2021/09/mckinsey-experts-offer-their-latest-analysis-on-when-covid-19-will-end/. Accessed 2 Aug 2021.

World Health Organization (WHO). (2020a). *Impact of COVID-19 on people's livelihoods, their health and our food systems.* https://www.who.int/news/item/13-10-2020-impact-of-covid-19-on-people%27s-livelihoods-their-health-and-our-food-systems. Accessed 1 Aug 2021.

World Health Organization (WHO). (2020b, May 4).*WHO Bangladesh COVID-19 situation report no 10.* https://www.who.int/docs/default-source/searo/bangladesh/covid-19-who-bangladesh-situation-reports/who-ban-covid-19-sitrep-10.pdf?sfvrsn=c0aac0b8_4. Accessed 5 Aug 2021.

Yadav, N. (2021). *These are the 10 most-affected countries with the highest number of COVID-19 cases.* https://www.businessinsider.in/politics/india/news/check-out-the-10-most-affected-countries-with-the-highest-number-of-coronavirus-cases/slidelist/76275918.cms

Yang, S. (2021, March 19). *Rising-power competition: The Covid-19 vaccine diplomacy of China and India.* The National Bureau of Asian Research. https://www.nbr.org/publication/rising-power-competition-the-covid-19-vaccine-diplomacy-of-china-and-india/. Accessed 4 Aug 2021.

Zhou, X., Snoswell, C. L., Harding, L. E., Bambling, M., Edirippulige, S., Bai, X., & Smith, A. C. (2020, Apr). The role of telehealth in reducing the mental health burden from COVID-19. *Telemedicine and e-Health, 26*(4), 377–379. https://doi.org/10.1089/tmj.2020.0068. Epub 2020 Mar 23. PMID: 32202977.

Uncited References

McKibbin, W., & Fernando, R. (2021). The global macroeconomic impacts of COVID-19: Seven scenarios. *Asian Economic Papers, 20*(2), 1–30.

Ullah, A. A., & Chattoraj, D. (2018). Roots of discrimination against Rohingya minorities: Society, ethnicity and international relations. *Intellectual Discourse, 26*(2), 541–565.

Ullah, A. A., Mohamad, S. M., Hassan, N. H., & Chattoraj, D. (2019). Global skills deficiency: Perspectives of skill mobility in Southeast Asian countries. *Asian Education and Development Studies, 8*(4), 416–432.

Printed in the United States
by Baker & Taylor Publisher Services